TAKE ME WITH YOU AND I WILL
CHANGE YOUR LIFE

TAKE ME WITH YOU AND I WILL CHANGE YOUR LIFE

THE MANNIELLO METHOD

The essential steps to achieve quality of life and longevity

Healthy habits – Food intolerances

Alternative medicines

Dr. DONATO MANNIELLO Ph.D.

CON EL PATROCINIO SIN FINES DE LUCRO DE

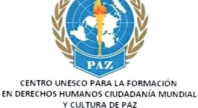

CENTRO UNESCO PARA LA FORMACIÓN
EN DERECHOS HUMANOS CIUDADANÍA MUNDIAL
Y CULTURA DE PAZ

Third edition: June 2019

© All rights reserved.

© Donato Alberto Manniello

Cover photography: © Fotolia.es

Interior design: © Germán Colli Lista

Interior photography: © Carolos Bell Ower and Antonio Belón M.

ISBN: 9781073345366

No part of this publication, including the cover design, may be reproduced, stored or transferred in any way or by any means, including electronically, chemically, mechanically, optically or by recording, in Internet or photocopy, without the previous permission from the publisher or the author. All rights reserved.

To my wife, lover and friend, Graciela, for being by my side at all times.

To my children, Margaux, Nathan, Estrella del Mar and Francesco, sources of strength in my life.

To my friends, Juan, Cristina, Poupée, Mónica Mario and Gastón, Marta and Sandro, for the precious time that they have shared with me.

To all those that have supported me in creating this book.

To the universe.

Content

Introduction	13
Chapter I - Healthy Habits	17
1. Healthy habits	19
Introduction	19
1.1. Healthy nutrition	27
1.1.1. A note on water	30
1.1.2. Breakfast	31
1.1.3. Advice on eating	34
1.1.3.1. What to avoid	34
- Coffee and its derivatives	34
- Chocolate and its derivatives	35
- Tobacco	35
- Alcohol	35
- Soft drinks and derivatives	37
- Artificial sweeteners	37
- Salt	37
- Raw tomato, honey, vinagre, lemon	38
- Orange juice in the morning	39
- Fried foods, cold cuts	39
- Dairy products	39
1.1.3.2. Calcium-rich foods	43
1.1.3.3. Foods to be avoided that contain dairy products	46
1.1.3.4. Plant-based drinks	47
1.1.3.5. More advice on eating	48
- How to shop	48
- How to cook	48
- How to store food	50
- Food storage time	52
- Frozen food storage time	54
1.1.4. Associations	56
1.1.4.1. Fermentation, putrefaction and consequences	58
1.1.4.2. Acid-base balance (pH)	59
- Causes of acid-base imbalance	60
- Effects of acid-base imbalances	61
- Treatment of acid-base imbalance	62
- List of acidifying foods	63
- List of alkalizing foods	64
1.1.4.3. Food groups	66
- Group 1: Vegetables	67
- Group 2: Carbohydrates	68
- Group 3: Legumes	69
- Group 4: Proteins	70
- Group 5: Fats	72
- Group 6: Fruits	73
1.1.4.4. Incorrect associations	75
- Association: Carbohydrates and proteins	75
- Association: Carbohydrates and acids	77

- Association: Carbohydrates and raw vegetables … 78
- Association: Carbohydrates and sugars … 79
- Association: Proteins and proteins … 80
- Association: Proteins and acids … 81
- Association: Proteins and fats … 83
- Association: Proteins and sugars … 85
- Summary … 86
1.1.4.5. Correct nutritional health guidelines … 88
- Summary of the food groups … 89
- Breakfast … 91
- Mid-morning … 91
- Lunch … 91
- Afternoon … 93
- Dinner … 93
- The application that will change your life … 94
- Recipes … 95
2. Physical health: Daily exercise … 108
2.1. Introduction … 109
2.2. Benefits of physical activity … 110
2.3. Waking up in the morning … 113
2.4. Walking 30 minutes a day … 123
2.5. Staying in shape … 125
2.5.1. Stretching … 125
2.5.2. Maintenance exercises … 133
2.6. Good posture habits … 143
3. Mental health: The positive mind … 145
3.1. Research findings … 145
3.2. The teachings of life … 146
3.3. Knowledge … 148
3.3.1. The pyramid … 149
3.3.2. The world of emotions … 151
3.3.3. The emotional boiling pots … 153
3.3.4. Behavior … 155
3.3.5. The freedom spiral … 156
3.4. Coincidences … 157
3.5. Excuses … 158
3.6. Creating your reality … 161
3.7. Recommendations … 163
3.7.1. Rejuvenate your brain … 163
3.7.2. Affirmations … 164
3.7.3. Avoid … 165
3.7.4. Personal life philosophy … 166
3.7.5. Personal peace … 168
3.7.6. Amaranta Method … 169

Chapter II - Food Intolerances … 171
1. Food intolerances … 173
1.1. What are intolerances? … 173
1.1.1. Intolerance and allergies, different concepts … 173
1.1.2. Additives: Preservatives and artificial coloring … 176
1.2. Do I have any food intolerances? … 178
1.3. Physiopathology of intolerances … 179

1.3.1. Intestinal dysbiosis	179
1.3.2. Functions of intestinal flora	179
1.3.3. Composition of intestinal flora	179
1.3.4. Causes of dysbiosis	180
1.3.5. Consequences of dysbiosis	181
1.3.6. Consequences of intestinal permeability	182
1.4. Symptoms associated with food intolerances	183
1.5. Treatment	185
1.5.1. Elimination of causes:	189
1.5.2. Cleansing of toxins.	190
1.5.3. Equilibrium of intestinal flora	190
1.5.4. Repair and protection of the intestinal membrane	191
1.5.5. Reintroduction of foods	191
1.5.6. Intake of nutrients for optimal absorption	192
Chapter III - Alternative Medicine	195
1. Introduction	197
1.1. Mechanical rebalancing	197
1.1.1. Osteopathy	197
1.1.2. Types of osteopathy	199
1.2. Energetic rebalancing	201
1.2.1. Traditional Chinese medicine	201
1.2.2. Acupuncture	203
1.2.3. Reiki	204
1.3. Functional rebalancing	207
1.3.1. Ayurvedic medicine	207
1.3.2. Connective tissue reflex therapy	209
1.3.2.1. Neural therapy principles	209
1.3.2.2. Means of action	210
1.4 Emotional rebalancing	212
1.4.1. Ericksonian therapeutic hypnosis	212
1.4.2 Brief Systemic Therapy	213
1.5. Complementary accompanying therapies	215
1.5.1. Phytotherapy	215
1.5.2. Nutritherapy or orthomolecular medicine	217
1.5.3. Homeopathy	219
1.5.4. Homeopathic mesotherapy	221
1.6. Essential oils and their effects in the daily life	223
1.6.1. What is an Essential Oil?	223
1.6.2. Essential Oils and Fatty Oils	225
1.6.3. The Limbic system	226
1.6.4. How Fragrance is Created	227
1.6.5. How fragrance is registered by the brain	227
1.6.6. Actions of essential oils	227
1.6.7. How to use them	228
1.6.8. « Raindrop Technique », a remarkable regimen for well-being	229
1.6.9. Some essentials oils and their properties	231
Chapter IV - Conclusions	233
Biography	239
Bibliography	241

INTRODUCTION

Each day we are more and more concerned about how we live and our well-being. Taking care of our health leads to a growing interest in different therapeutic means.

Current issues commonly affecting health today include excessive weight, obesity, major risk pathologies (diabetes, hypertension, etc.), depression, education, multinational food and pharmaceutical companies...

We can easily say that these issues are problems of our society, but we must also recognize that they are our own problems on a personal level and that we are the ones that responsible for our choices.

We choose to eat a certain food or not, we choose to exercise or not, we choose how we think, and we even choose to take a medication or not.

We must recognize and take into account that the decision is always our own.

The patient, who is currently tired of excessive medication, looks for alternatives to their medical problems, and this is why alternative medicines are in clear expansion, without overlooking the fact that these have existed for more than five thousand years.

We are already frequently using techniques that have been around for thousands of years such as osteopathy, acupuncture, medicinal herbs, diet, exercise, meditation, etc., to treat different maladies and disorders.

After many years of experience in various therapeutic fields and more than twenty years of research on food and nutrition, I have developed a simple and effective method that is accessible to everyone that wishes to have great quality of life, in all aspects: mechanical, energetic, functional and emotional.

My experience tells me that the patient should be treated as a whole: with mechanical, energetic, functional and emotional rebalancing. My therapeutic concept consists of the use of several different therapies.

This book will explain the essential steps to achieve a healthy life. It is not about adding on years of life, but healthy life to the years.

Keep in mind that the success of these therapies is based on a meticulous and holistic diagnosis of the patient as an individual, taking into account his or her life habits (eating, work, family, etc.).

I would like to thank you for your interest in healthy habits and alternative medicine, and I hope that you can find here the information that you need to incorporate them into your daily life.

Dr. Donato Manniello, Ph.

"The art of manual therapy is ancient. I greatly esteem those that discovered it, as well as those that by several generations succeed me and whose work contributes to the development of the natural art of curing".

HIPPOCRATES, 435 b.C.

CHAPTER I

HEALTHY HABITS

1. HEALTHY HABITS

INTRODUCTION

In 21st century society, obesity has reached epidemic proportions worldwide, and each year at least 3.4 million people die due to obesity or overweight, which is why it is considered a health problem that must be addressed.

Although previously considered a problem confined to high-income countries, obesity is now also prevalent in low- and middle-income countries.

WHO places the blame for the escalation in obesity on the price of healthier foods for the poorest families and societies.

A study carried out by the World Health Organization (WHO) and Imperial College London on the occasion of World Obesity Day predicts that, if the trend continues, in 2022 the number of children and adolescents (between five and 19 years) with obesity will exceed those who are moderately or severely underweight. Today there are 10 times more children and adolescents with obesity than 40 years ago. The study analyzed 130 million boys and girls between 1975 and 2016.

Thus, they have seen how obesity rates have gone from 1% in 1975 to 6% and 8% in girls and boys respectively in 2016. In figures, it has gone from 11 to 124 million children and adolescents with obesity.

Governments, international partners, civil society, non-governmental organizations and the private sector all play a crucial role in the prevention of obesity.

Important information to keep in mind:

. In 2016, more than 1,900 million adults were overweight and more than 650 million were obese.

.In 2016, 41 million children under the age of five were overweight worldwide. These children are very likely to become obese adults who are more likely to suffer from diabetes and cardiovascular disease at an early age, and of course premature death and disability.

. The support of the community and the environment are fundamental to influencing personal choices and avoiding obesity. We must mobilize to inform people about the healthiest dietary options.

. The choices of children, their diet and the habit of doing physical activities depend on the environment around them. That is why it is essential to keep repeating that a healthy diet and regular physical activity can help prevent obesity.

The obesity rate has doubled in Spain in the last 20 years; currently it is estimated that more than half of the adult population, 53%, is overweight, 36% of the population as a whole is overweight and 17% is obese.

In the case of children, 12% are overweight and 14% are obese.

The OECD (Organization for Economic Cooperation and Development) has just published the Obesity Update 2017 report (Update on obesity 2017) in order to show the current situation of the so-called epidemic of the 21st century. It shows in which countries it has increased, has remained stable or reduced, which age groups and gender it affects most, what policies and strategies are being implemented to deal with obesity, the predicted increase in its prevalence, etc.

This report shows the ranking of OECD countries with the highest rate of obesity, and although it is now being presented, it must be said that the data have been analyzed up to 2015. If the data were current, some figures would probably be different, because during the last two years the fight to stop the rise in the obesity rate has intensified. According to the data, at 38.2%, the United States leads the classification of the adult population (over 15 years) with the highest rate of obesity, followed by Mexico with 32.4% and New Zealand with 30.7%. .

At the other extreme, we find the countries with the lowest rate of obesity in the adult population. Japan leads this classification with only 3.7%, followed by Korea with 5.3% and Italy with 9.8%. According to the report, during the last five years the obesity rate has continued to grow, although at a slower pace than in previous years. The average rate of overweight and obesity in the OECD countries is set at 19.5% of the adult population and 17% of the child population. However, the rate of increase is expected to continue to slow steadily until the year 2030.

Many of the actions being implemented focus on trying to raise awareness among the population of the importance of following a healthy lifestyle and diet. The report highlights actions such as recommending the consumption of seven servings of fruits and vegetables per day, or the use of social networks to carry out promotional campaigns to improve health. It is considered that nutrition can be improved through communication.

The Lancet magazine has published in its latest edition a study, The Global Burden of Disease, in which it demonstrates the deadly consequences of an unbalanced diet. Eating badly kills one in five people in the world: the lethal weapon of poor diet. In 2017, 11 million people died worldwide from diseases related to an unbalanced diet. This is almost ten times more than the deaths in the same period caused by traffic accidents. The authors analyze the consumption of 15 types of foods in 195 countries between 1990 and 2017. They conclude that a high number of deaths are associated with not following a healthy diet.

Inappropriate nutrition caused ten million people to die from cardiovascular diseases, 913,000 from cancer and 339,000 from type 2 diabetes. The figures are even more worrying if we consider that deaths from these causes have increased by three million in only 29 years.

The WHO has recommended reducing the daily salt consumption of 5 grams daily to 2. But salt is taken in excess, twice as much as recommended. Such a basic and cheap seasoning is one of the biggest causes of death from cardiovascular diseases.

As for sugar-sweetened beverages -another of the big culprits of excess mortality- people ingest 10 times more than they should. The typical can of 330 milliliters contains neither more nor less than 35 grams of sugar and the WHO recommends a maximum daily consumption of added sugars of 25 grams.

A researcher at the University of Washington, Christopher Murray, points out: "This study affirms what many have thought for several years: that a poor diet is responsible for more deaths than any other risk factor in the world." Therefore there is an urgent need to make food policies that promote balanced diets, adds the expert.

People that are obese at 40 years old can lose up to 7 years of their life according to the latest research. The WHO (World Health Organization) has started a campaign against childhood obesity considering it as one of the principal threats to public health. Within the campaign, dietary guidelines will be created, interventions will be designed to be carried out in schools to promote and reinforce physical activity, the food and drinks available at the schools will be evaluated, recommendations will be made to the industry geared toward modifying the composition of foods to reduce their fat, sugar and salt content, especially in the case of the bread that is consumed in Spain, that presents salt levels that are above the European average, and the areas of research and treatment of obesity and eating disorders will also be analyzed.

The less we eat, the longer we live. The reduction of calories is directly proportional to longevity. This theory has been demonstrated with monkeys: after studying them for more than 20 years, it was confirmed that if they ate less, they lived longer and presented less cases of cancer, diabetes, fewer cardiovascular problems or cerebral atrophy.

What we eat also makes us age: the presence of nutrients in foods has been decreasing over the last several years. Fast food and other recently created synthetic foods limit our longevity and deteriorate the quality of our aging process. Not only must we eat less, but we must give our organisms the high quality nutrients necessary to avoid any deficiencies.

The principal causes of these high levels of obesity are changes in eating habits (unhealthy diets) and lack of physical activity. "An average of 19% more calories than those needed are consumed and there is not enough physical activity to burn this excess off", claims Elena Salgado.

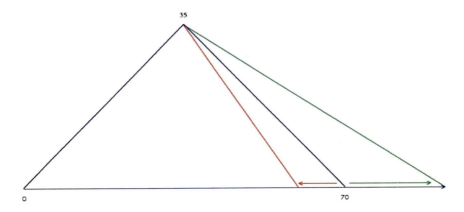

From our birth until approximately the age of 35 to 36 years, everything seems to function perfectly. However, after this age, we begin to feel the effects of the aging process. If we do not already have healthy habits, we will reduce our life span, and, on the contrary, if we do, we will be able to lengthen our life span, enjoying great health.

When we talk about longevity, we have to keep in mind our genetics. Taking care of our DNA and its telomeres is fundamental. Each chromosome (we have 24 pairs in each cell) is the manner in which our DNA is organized, together with proteins, within the nucleus of our cells. A chromosome is one single molecule of DNA, which contains many genes (fragments with information) and other regulating elements.

The telomeres are specialized chromatin structures that are found located on the ends of the chromosome arms. They seem to be implicated in numerous cellular functions, especially those related with the control of the duration of life on a cellular level.

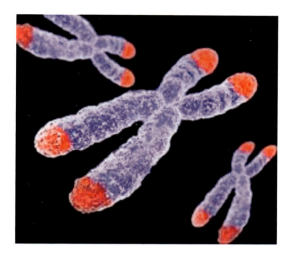

Chromosomes in violet and telomeres in red.

These telomeres protect the genetic information and help the DNA to replicate more easily to allow for new cellular divisions. Every time that a cell divides, its telomeres are shortened. They are like a marker of cell age: with each year lived, more cellular divisions take place and the telomeres become shorter.

When the telomeres reach a specific minimum size, the cells stop functioning and become incapable of participating in the normal functions of the tissue where they are located. This could play an important role in the overall aging of the entire organism.

We should also highlight the fact that the telomeres protect our genes. When the size of the telomeres is reduced, our genetic material is less protected, increasing the risk of mutations in the chromosomes and, therefore, favoring the possibility of having different cancers in the future.

According to the above-mentioned, an adequate diet protects our DNA and its corresponding telomeres, thus lengthening our lives and providing better quality of life.

I will later explain how orthomolecular medicine aids in genetic repair, protecting DNA and keeping telomeres active for better health and quality of life.

My professional experience has shown me that the three most important pillars are:

- HEALTHY NUTRITION
- PHYSICAL HEALTH: DAILY EXERCISE
- MENTAL HEALTH: POSITIVE MIND

"A wise man must consider that his health is the greatest of human blessings"

(Hippocrates)

1.1. HEALTHY NUTRITION

When we ingest foods, we intake calories (energy) into our body. We are constantly told that if we intake more than we burn, that is, if we have eat more calories than those that our body can use, we will get fat. And, on the contrary, if we burn more energy than what we consume, we will lose weight, as we will be under the energy levels needed for the correct functioning of our body.

Just as the computer at our bank analyzes the fluctuations of our account balance, our organism analyzes and memorizes the deposits and withdrawals of calories. This way, when there is a period of few deposits, for example, when following one of the many "miracle diets" in order to lose weight quickly before summer, our organism activates an energetic deficit alarm.

If after a period of time, the normal amount of deposits is once again made, when abandoning the useless diet, the bank (organism), foreseeing future periods of energetic crisis, adopts a savings and maximum profitability plan for its calories, achieving a rapid increase in its level of fats, surpassing previous levels in many cases.

According to the World Health Organization (WHO), being overweight means carrying an excess of all types of body tissues: fatty mass and fat-free mass (muscles, bones and water). Obesity is a physical state of excessive body fat.

Body Mass Index (BMI)

The body mass index (BMI) relates weight with height, as expressed in the following formula. This index has the advantage of using two variables that are easily measured and very precise.

BMI = weight (Kg) / height (m)2

For example, for a person that weighs 70 kg and is 1.60 meters tall, their BMI would be 70 / 1.602, that is, 27.3, a value that according to the WHO would correspond with overweight or class I obesity.

Classification of obesity based on BMI according to the WHO:

NORMAL WEIGHT	18.5 – 24.9
OVERWEIGHT (OBESE CLASS I)	25 – 29.9
PRE-OBESITY (OBESE CLASS II)	30 – 34.9
OBESITY (OBSESE CLASS III)	35 – 39.9
MORBID OBESITY (OBESE CLASS IV)	> 40

When people talk about a healthy diet, they are almost always referring to the "Mediterranean diet". It is one of the best philosophies of a healthy life style based on a diet composed of a combination of different traditional ingredients. It is a way to try to recover a more traditional food system and adapt it to a social system of nutritional practices and habits. The combination of its elements contributes to the creation of a healthy diet.

Nutrition in the fetal period, childhood and adolescence of an individual ensures their growth takes place with all of the individual's genetic possibilities.

Different studies have demonstrated that between populations exposed to the same environmental influences (climate, temperature, housing, etc.), different dietary habits determine clear differences regarding physical development and

that of the character of the population and the illnesses that they suffer.

Thus, those civilizations with a diet that has a mixed and varied base are more physically and psychologically developed. Also, they show better overall health than those populations with strictly vegetarian customs or, on the contrary, strictly meat-based diets, etc.

In the Mediterranean, differences are still found in the height and weight of children from families of different economic levels, which clearly suggests that these differences are established based on the different diets that they receive.

It seems clear that the period of life from the fetus to 5 years old is a critical stage in the growth and development of an individual. It has been demonstrated that a delay suffered in this period from a deficit of nutrients is hard to overcome, even if the individual later receives an adequate diet.

Therefore, diet in children is one of the primordial causes of the existence of differences regarding physical and mental development, independent of the individual limitations from genetic inheritance, hygiene or physical activity.

Definitively, we must reduce the intake of calories by 20 to 30%, avoid fast food, provide the organism with the necessary nutrients and correctly associate foods – which I will later explain -. These are good recommendations to make our diets healthier.

1.1.1. A NOTE ON WATER

Water is life!

Without water, no life is possible on earth. Men, animals, plants and food contain water. A newborn baby is made up of 85% water and an elderly person still possesses 60%.

The transportation of substances needed for the organism to function through blood and lymphatic fluids is possible thanks to water. It is the medium where the greatest portion of metabolic reactions takes place and it ensures the elimination of a large portion of metabolic waste (urine, transpiration, feces…).

The role of water is fundamental in all mechanisms of life. Hydration of the organism should thus be continuous. We should not wait until we are thirsty to drink water. Actually, when a person is thirsty, there is already a high level of dehydration.

Drinking water first thing in the morning is currently popular in Japan. For older people with illnesses, water treatment has been successful for the Japanese medical society, with a curing rate of 100% for the following diseases: headaches, arthritis, excess weight, bronchitis, urinary and kidney diseases, vomiting, gastritis, diarrhea, hemorrhoids, constipation, menstrual disorders, and ear, nose and throat diseases among others.

Chinese and Japanese people drink hot tea with their meals instead of cold water. It is nice to drink a glass of cold water during or after meals, however, cold drinks solidify the fats that you have just eaten. This slows digestion.

Drinking two liters of water per day, away from meals, to avoid diluting gastric juices that are necessary for proper digestion, is recommended for all of the above-mentioned reasons.

1.1.2. BREAKFAST

"A hungry stomach will not allow its owner to ignore it, in spite of his or her many concerns and worries"

(Homer, VIII century BC)

For those that do not have breakfast saying that food doesn't sit well at that time of day:

The word BREAKFAST means "BREAKING THE FAST".

From the moment we finish dinner to the moment we wake up the next day, 8 to 10 hours (or more) have passed. Our factory (organism) has been working all night, consuming all of the energy provided at dinner. If we don't provide any raw material in the morning, the factory cannot produce the final product (energy).

WHY HAVE BREAKFAST?

The first good reason to have breakfast is the healthy benefits that we receive. The second is the damage that we cause in our body by fasting in the morning. This is what takes place in our organism when we do not eat breakfast: the alarm clock goes off and our brain starts to worry: "It's time to get up and we have already burned all of our fuel". The first neuron available is called upon to send a message to see how much glucose is available in the bloodstream. A response comes back from the blood saying "there is enough sugar here for about 15 – 20 minutes, at most". The brain makes a doubtful gesture and says to the messenger neuron "ok, talk to the liver and find out what he's got stored away".

The savings account is checked in the liver and the liver responds that "at most, the funds can cover 20 – 25 minutes". There is a total of close to 290 grams of glucose, that is, enough to cover 45 minutes of activity. During this time, the brain is begging us to have breakfast.

If we are in a hurry or we cannot stand eating in the morning, the brain will have to sound the necessary alarms: "maximum alert: forced economy. CORTISONE will take glucose from muscle cells, ligaments, bones and collagen from skin". The cortisone will start up the mechanisms for the cells to open up and release their proteins. These proteins will then travel to the liver to be transformed into blood glucose. The process will continue until we eat again.

As you can see, people who do not eat breakfast are tricking themselves: what really happens is that they eat their own muscles, they devour themselves. Consequently, they lose muscular tone, and their brain, instead of taking care of intellectual functions, spends the entire morning activating the emergency system to obtain fuel and food.

HOW DOES THIS AFFECT OUR WEIGHT?

When we start the day fasting, an energy-saving strategy is triggered and the metabolism thus decreases. The brain does not know if the fasting will last for a few hours or a few days and it therefore takes the most severe measures.

This way, if the person decides to later have lunch or a mid-morning snack, it will be accepted as extra and will be directed towards the "fat reserves" storage and the person will gain weight.

The muscles are the first to be used as a fuel reserve during morning fasting because the cortisol or hydrocortisone is the dominant hormone at this time. They stimulate the destruction of muscle proteins and their conversion into glucose.

We also must not fall into the saying that we must "eat like a king in the morning, like a prince at midday and like a beggar at dinner". If you eat too much in the morning, your stomach will expand and then ask for greater quantities of food later. The healthiest option is to always "eat like a prince".

We must provide the factory (our organism) with raw material in order to obtain a continuous energy source. Five meals a day is the ideal (this will be explained later).

"If we could give all individuals the proper quantity of food and exercise, not too much or too little, we would have found the safest path to good health"

(Hippocrates)

1.1.3. ADVICE ON EATING

1.1.3.1. WHAT TO AVOID

- COFFEE AND ITS DERIVATIVES

The excessive consumption of coffee (more than 1 cup a day) is detrimental to our health. Its action against sleeping is a know effect of coffee although possible insomnia can be avoided by moderate intake and not having any in the afternoon and evening.

Various studies have shown the relationship between the consumption of coffee and various illnesses, from diabetes and cardiovascular diseases to cancer and cirrhosis.

Likewise, caffeine has been identified as an irritant to the digestive system and people who suffer from, or have a history of, gastritis or peptic ulcers, both at the gastric and duodenal levels, should thus avoid it.

Coffee also has a strong diuretic effect and those with kidney problems should also avoid it as it makes the kidneys work even harder.

Our pH is acidified by the consumption of coffee favoring the demineralization of our organism. It invariably produces in all cases nervous alterations due to its properties. Certain neurological alterations prohibit its use in certain patients due to its effects that directly attack the central nervous system.

When I talk about coffee derivatives I am referring to mixtures that are harmful to the stomach. The worst combination is drinking coffee with milk or cream, associated with any type of sugars (refined, white, raw or chemically transformed sugars – saccharine, aspartame, etc.).

Try savoring a cup of coffee without adding sugar or milk, enjoying its aroma and strong flavor…but just one.

We know that our body, when he is in a good health, he has a frequency measured in Megahertz that varies between 62 MHz and 68 MHz. The disease begins to settle when the energy goes down to 58 MHz. The symptoms of the flu begin at 57 MHz. Candida installs at 55 MHz. The herpes virus manifests at 52 MHz and the cancer at 42 MHz.

Now, when we only take the coffee cup, in 3 seconds the energy goes down to 58 MHz. And when we drink a sip of coffee the frequency goes down in 3 seconds to 52 MHz. Afterwards the body takes 3 days to return to the normal.

- CHOCOLATE AND ITS DERIVATIVES

Cacao contains many important substances such as anandamide, arginine, dopamine (neurotransmitter), epicatechin (antioxidant), histamines, magnesium, serotonin (neurotransmitter), tryptophan (essential to trigger the liberation of the serotonin neurotransmitter), phenethylamine, polyphenols (antioxidants), tyramine, salsolinol and flavonoids.

Its stimulating effect is due to a substance called theobromine, which produces an increase of the levels of serotonin and dopamine. Cacao-based products that contain sugar can intensify this stimulating effect by increasing the levels of serotonin and dopamine even more. Black chocolate made of 70% pure cacao can be consumed. Under this percentage of pure cacao (milk chocolate, chocolate with fruit, with nuts, etc.), significant quantities of sugar and fats are added and it should be avoided.

- TOBACCO

I do not believe it is necessary to talk about the problems tobacco produces...its clearly written on the packaging: SMOKING KILLS!!

- ALCOHOL

Alcohol, aside from being an addictive drug, is the cause of 60 different diseases and ailments, including liver and pancreas damage, mental and behavioral disorders, gastrointestinal problems, cancer, cardiovascular, lung and musculoskeletal diseases, reproductive disorders as well as prenatal damage, a greater risk of premature labor and low birth weight.

One of the principal conclusions of a study titled "Alcohol in Europe: a public health perspective", created by the Institute of Alcohol Studies, in the United Kingdom, concludes that "alcohol increases the risk of disease exponentially; greater consumption leads to greater risk".

Alcohol does not affect everyone in the same manner. Women's metabolism is different than that of men. Women weigh less, their constitution is smaller and their organism contains less water. This means that their tolerance to alcohol is lower.

Generally speaking, under 30 grams of alcohol per day is a safe amount, from 30 to 60 grams of alcohol daily is of moderate risk and more than 60 grams of alcohol daily is considered high risk (for the risk of cirrhosis).

The grams of alcohol are calculated by multiplying the degree of alcohol found in the drink, which are grams of alcohol per every 100 cc, multiplied by the quantity, divided by 100. For example:

- A bottle (750 cc) of red wine (usually with a 12% degree of alcohol) will have 750 x 12 / 100 = 90 grams;
- 4 glasses (250 cc) of normal beer (5%) will have 4 x 250 x 5 / 100 = 50 grams.;
- 2 glasses (125 cc) of whisky (40%) will have 100 grams of alcohol…

- SOFT DRINKS AND DERIVATIVES (TONIC WATER, ZERO, ETC.)

Knowing that the quantity of sugars added not only increases the overload of calories in the organism, but that we will trigger the formation of kidney stones and prepare ourselves for diabetes in the future.

- ARTIFICIAL SWEETENERS (SACCHARINE, ASPARTAME, ETC.)

It has been proven that chemically transformed sugars can cause cardiovascular problems. "Sugar-free" drinks are full of these artificial sweeteners. The use of fructose or stevia is recommended to avoid any problems. Stevia is a plant that has been used for thousands of years by South American tribes, primarily in Paraguay, Bolivia and Argentina, and that can be up to 300 times sweeter than common sugar, with low amounts of carbohydrates and sugars. Its possible benefits in the treatment of obesity and high blood pressure have been demonstrated.

- SALT

Common salt, or what we simply call "salt", is made up of a salt called sodium chloride whose chemical formula is NaCl. There are four types of salt, according to their origin: sea salt and spring salt (that is obtained through evaporation); rock salt, which comes from the mining of a mineral rock known as halite; and vegetable salt, that is obtained through concentration, by boiling the gramineae plant.

Salt (common salt) is a condiment that improves or strengthens flavors and that is also a great source of essential nutrients, fundamentally, sodium and chloride.

Salt can be found in many forms although the most common is the sodium-type, that is, salt composed by sodium chloride in a ratio of 4:6. We must highlight that potassium chloride also exists.

Our organism uses salt for several different functions: to form hydrochloric acid that is found in the stomach; constructing hematic or blood parts; regulating muscular processes; and forming part of the extracellular fluid. As a fundamental benefit, I will highlight the fact that it satisfies the basic metabolic needs for sodium in the organism while stabilizing blood pressure.

It is also a great preservative, impeding or complicating the appearance of microorganisms that decompose or deteriorate foods.

At the same time, salt must be consumed with moderation (between 2 and 4 grams per day) as the excess or absence of sodium can have harmful effects on our health.

High blood pressure, or hypertension, is one of the inconveniences of the excessive intake of salt. It is a risk factor for later developing cardiovascular diseases, stomach diseases, asthmatic problems, loss of calcium or osteoporosis, and, together with an excess of calcium, the appearance of kidney and gallstones.

The deficiency of salt can cause symptoms of apathy, weakness, fainting, anorexia, low blood pressure, circulatory collapse, shock and even death.

Ultimately, although it can be a nutritional complement, I highly recommend moderating salt intake due to the risk of affecting your health in the above mentioned ways. If you already have been diagnosed with high blood pressure, make sure you limit your intake of the sodium that is found in the composition of foods that we eat on a daily basis, and you should moderate the consumption of those foods that we know have a higher sodium concentration.

- RAW TOMATO, HONEY, VINAGRE, LEMON

Acids and sugars produce a delay in the secretion of chloric acid which inhibits all digestion, especially that of proteins. These foods should not be eaten with meals.

- ORANGE JUICE IN THE MORNING

After fasting (before breakfast), along with affixing fats in the organism, oranges produce significant fermentation that produces alcohol. We all know about the consequences of alcohol on the liver, pancreas and the other disorders it can cause.

- FRIED FOODS, COLD CUTS

The presence of fat in foods reduces gastric secretions, the quantity of enzymes and weakens gastric tone by 50%. This inhibitory effect can last two or more hours.

- DAIRY PRODUCTS

It is known that after a certain age, approximately 7 years old, that we no longer produce the enzymes necessary to digest milk (lactase and renin). However, this does vary by race and the percentage of people that have dairy intolerances is extremely high in Africa and Asia, and somewhat less, due to a mutation, in Europe and the Americas. That said, and in spite of it, we are recommended to consume dairy products daily, with the justification that our calcium needs will be met for proper growth and maintenance of our bones.

How could something that cannot be digested be good for our health? What does the baby calf do when it stops drinking its mother's milk? It eats grass!

Human beings are the only mammals that drink milk that comes from other animals once they have grown out of the breastfeeding period. The milk that is produced by each mammal is ideal for its species and not others.

Many nutritionists recommend milk as a good source of calcium, arguing that it is indispensable for bone health. Many people adhere to this recommendation and consume large quantities of milk. Millions of North Americans drink milk instead of water.

However, it is precisely in the United States, the world's milk consumer, where there is a higher rate of osteoporosis than in any other place. What a paradox! Jane E. Kerstetten and Lindsay H. Allen reach the conclusion that the intake of calcium and phosphorous consumed by adults in America, by increasing the amount of proteins in their diet, increases the presence of calcium in urine, leading to a negative difference in the calcium balance. In other words, more calcium is eliminated from the body by urine when we consume animal proteins in the form of dairy products (milk, yogurt, cheese), and even eggs and chicken. The amount of calcium in milk is one thing, but its bioavailability is another altogether.

The China study, by Dr. T. Colin Campdell, shows that animal milk acidifies our organism and demineralizes our bones, which can cause osteoporosis.

Thanks to research done by Dr. John McDougall, it is known that "the African Bantu woman is an excellent example of good health. Her diet is dairy-free and provides her with 250 to 400 mg of calcium from plant sources, which is what half of Western women intake. Bantu women have an average of ten babies during their life and they breastfeed all of them for approximately ten months…Osteoporosis is relatively absent among these women".

Dr. Jean Seignalet tells us that "cow's milk has a number of disadvantages for humans. Cow's milk and its derivatives are forbidden: butter, cheese, cream, icecream, yogurt, etc. Animal's milk should be removed from our diets, regardless of its origin: cow, goat, sheep, horse…"

And what about casein?

A breastfeeding child assimilates casein well from his or her mother's milk, but not from cow's milk. An allergy to casein triggers the liberation of chemical products such as histamines that cause symptoms such as:

- Swelling of lips, mouth, throat, face...
- Skin reactions, cutaneous rashes, hives, redness, itchiness...
- and pulmonary congestion...

It is also good to know that milk contains 59 types of hormones (pituitary, corticosteroids, adrenal, sexual...) that can be the cause of diverse degenerative diseases. Among said hormones, the growth hormone (IGF-1) is especially important, whose action, together with the proteins found in cow's milk, enables the rapid growth of calves so that they double their weight in a very short amount of time. It is also evident that this is not a necessity for humans. High levels of this hormone, together with other toxins, are considered today as a nutrition-related source of cancer.

"The medicine world reports that the IGF-1 is the principal factor of growth and proliferation of cancer in breasts, ovaries, uterus, prostate, colon, etc. and it is suspected to be the base of all types of cancers".

I must add that milk can be contaminated by chemical products, hormones, antibiotics, pesticides, pus from mastitis – frequent in cows that are continuously milked-, virus, bacteria, etc.

In fact, the consumption of milk and its derivatives has been associated with iron deficiency anemia, rheumatoid arthritis, osteoarthritis, asthma, autism, cataracts, colitis ulcerosa, type 1 diabetes, abdominal pain, Crohn's disease, coronary diseases, multiple sclerosis, constipation, chronic fatigue, anal fistulae and fissures, urinary incontinence or enuresis, migraine headaches, ear and throat conditions, sinusitis, allergic reactions, malabsorption syndrome, sleeping disorders, peptic ulcers, acidosis, learning difficulties in children, female infertility, lymphomas and with cancer of the stomach, breast, ovary, uterus, prostate, testicle, and pancreas.

"The arteries of children that have several glasses of milk every day are in worse condition than those that have no milk".

There are several lines of research that show that health improves notably when milk and its derivatives are removed from a person's diet. Here are two examples:

- People that suffer from osteoarthritis and/or arthritis and stop consuming dairy products (milk, yogurt, dairy-based beverages, fresh cheeses…), experience a 70% reduction of pain.

- Children that suffer from colds, stuffy noses, or chronic mucus-producing bronchitis that stop consuming dairy products return to having good health.

"The reality is that there are many milk cows, and please, don't waste their milk. It can be sold for great amounts of money!" This is one of the principal reasons that milk is said to be so healthy. Tons of money is invested daily on the publicity for dairy products, for both adults and children, all while the harmful effects of milk are readily known. It is surprising that the dairy industry has been able to spread its message to such a great degree.

Do you remember Popeye the Sailor Man? He told us that if we ate spinach, full of iron, we would be as strong as him. During the great depression in the United States there was mass production of spinach that nobody wanted to consume…and what happened? Popeye was a simple political invention to convince people to consume spinach. Did you know that there is hardly any iron in spinach?

The same thing happened with dairy products, deceptive

advertising, that only talked about the benefits and not the negative effects.

The million dollar question: why do we consume dairy products?

The million dollar answer: to have calcium for our bones!!

The reality is that we can obtain calcium from many different sources. It is abundant in the soil and a sufficient amount can be obtained from vegetables, legumes, salads and fruit. A comparative list of the percentage of calcium in different types of food is shown below.

Professor Henri Joyeux, doctor and oncologist, tells us: "Too much calcium is like at the bottom of the kettle. At the intestinal level too much calcium will act as an irritant, producing polyps, cysts, stones and calcifications of all kinds" and even cancer. There are 7 growth factors in breast milk, 7 neurotrophic factors for the brain. In cow's milk there are 3:1 factor for the skin, 1 factor for the bones and joints and 1 factor for insulin for the digestive tract. These 3 factors are responsible for 25% of cancers. The dairy products of large animals are the cause of autoimmune diseases.

Cow's milk has 4 times more calcium than human milk. Calcium enters the blood and reaches the bone ... and the bone tells it that it does not want it because it has everything it needs, and it goes elsewhere! It will enter into the sinuses, ovaries, prostate..., causing micro calcifications with a risk of cancer. It will enter the joints and cause all kinds of osteoarthritis, arthritis...

The women who consume the most milk products in the world are in Sweden, and these are the ones that have the most osteoporosis! "

1.1.3.2. CALCIUM-RICH FOODS

Remember that cow's milk has 120 mg of calcium per 100 gr edible serving.

	CALCIO/100 gr
Soy milk, oat milk	120 mg.
Egg yoke	130 mg.

VEGETABLES

Swiss chard	113 mg
Watercress	170 mg
Cardoon, leek	115 mg
Parsley	200 mg
Spinach	87 mg
Celery, green beans, lettuce	60 mg
Artichoke, cabbage, kale, string beans, carrot, onion, radish	40 mg

LEGUMES

Garbanzos, chickpeas	145 mg
Dried broad beans	115 mg
Beans (white, pinto, etc.)	128 mg
Lentils	56 mg

GRAINS

Oats, barley, rye	60 mg
Whole wheat, brown rice	50 mg
Wheat	40 mg

FRUITS

Kiwi	56 mg
Lemon	45 mg
Strawberries	30 mg
Oranges	28 mg
Grapes	20 mg
Cherries, mango, plum	18 mg
Apple, banana, pear	12 mg
Melon, peach	10 mg

NUTS AND DRIED FRUITS

Almonds	254 mg
Hazelnuts	192 mg
Dried figs	178 mg
Pistachios	136 mg
Walnuts	70 mg
Dates	70 mg

SEAFOOD

FRESH FISH, SHELLFISH AND CRUSTACEANS
Clams, baby clams, cockles	128 mg
Snails	140 mg
Crawfish, prawns, shrimp	220 mg
Oysters, scallops, goose barnacles	130 mg
Octopus	145 mg
Sole	120 mg
Sardines	98 mg
Cod	51 mg

CANNED SEAFOOD
Sardines in oil	400 mg
Clams, cockles and similar	128 mg

Recommendation from health authorities for the daily consumption of calcium :

Up to 6 months of age	400 mg
Between 6 and 12 months	600 mg
Between 1 and 10 years	800 mg
Between 11 and 24 years	1,5 gr
Pregnant and breastfeeding women	1,5 gr
Women between 25 and 50 years	1 / 1,5 gr
Women between 51 and 65 years	1 / 1,5 gr
Men between 25 and 65 years	1 / 1,5 gr

1.1.3.3. FOODS TO BE AVOIDED THAT CONTAIN DAIRY PRODUCTS

There are many ready-made meals that may contain cow's milk. If it appears in the list of ingredients on the label, the meal should be avoided.

- WHOLE, 2% AND NONFAT OR SKIM MILK, POWDERED MILK, CONDENSED MILK, BUTTERMILK AND DULCE DE LECHE.
- YOGURT AND CREAM.
- FRESH CHEESES, COTTAGE CHEESE AND CHEESE CURD.
- ICECREAM, SORBET AND MILKSHAKES.
- PUDDING, PROFITEROLES, SOUFFLES, CREPES, PANCAKES AND WAFFLES.
- CHOCOLATE, CHOCOLATE DRINKS.
- CUSTARD, FLAN, RICE PUDDING.
- WHITE SAUCES, BECHAMEL.
- CERTAIN BATTERS FOR FRYING.
- MASHED POTATOES.
- CERTAIN PASTRIES/SWEETS (cakes, cookies, tea biscuits, donuts).
- CERTAIN BREADS (ready-sliced bread).
- WHEY, LACTASE.
- SALAD DRESSING AND MANY TYPES OF SAUCES.
- CERTAIN EGG DISHES.
- SAUSAGES AND COLD CUTS (sliced ham, pork shoulder, sliced turkey, salami…).

1.1.3.4. PLANT-BASED DRINKS: HEALTHY ALTERNATIVES TO MILK

Having a good alternative to milk is a good idea. Soymilk is well known, but there are numerous other plant-based drinks that are available:

- Soymilk or beverage.
- Oat milk or beverage.
- Rice milk or beverage.
- Almond milk or beverage.
- Hazelnut milk or beverage.
- Horchata (tigernut).
- Chestnut milk or beverage (powder).
- Walnut milk or beverage (powder).
- Quinoa milk or beverage (liquid and powder).
- Spelt milk or beverage (liquid and powder).
- Kamut grain milk or beverage (liquid).
- Millet milk or beverage (liquid).
- Sesame milk or beverage (powder).

In some cases, there are more dense versions to substitute cream used for cooking.

NOTE

Soymilk can be boiled for 25 minutes over a low flame, with lemon zest (thoroughly washed), cinnamon or vanilla. Once cooled, it can be kept in a covered bottle and stored in the refrigerator for a delicious and refreshing beverage.

1.1.3.5. MORE ADVICE ON EATING TO MAXIMIZE NUTRIENT UPTAKE

- HOW TO SHOP

When possible, always buy fresh foods that have not been processed.

- Eat biologically cultivated foods.
- Buy local, seasonal produce.
- Store food in a fresh, dark place.
- Consume food as soon as possible after purchasing.
- Wash fruits and vegetables thoroughly.
- Peel any fruits or vegetables that may have been treated with pesticides.
- Do not buy produce packaged in Styrofoam.
- And if there is no other option, remove them immediately once at home and store them in a clean recipient, preferably glass.

- HOW TO COOK

Our metabolism is programed from the beginning of time to accept and dissolve natural and raw foods through digestion. Research has been conducted on the effect that heat produces on foods that demonstrates that various new molecules appear, in some cases up to 450. Also, keep in mind that when we cook we almost always use more than one kind of food…

Each time that we introduce strange foreign molecules into our digestive tract, due to the lack of digestive enzymes for said molecules, these are not broken down or used by our metabolism. This happens as a consequence of the "biochemical confusion" caused in our body by cooking food.

When cooking vegetables, the following are lost into the water used for cooking:

- 40 to 60% of minerals.
- 95% of vitamins and bases.

The importance of the Asian system of steaming vegetables in steel or bamboo baskets, without any direct contact with water, comes from these facts. The water from boiling or steaming vegetables preserves the high alkaline content of the cooked vegetables and has a high therapeutic value.

After providing the previous information, I would also like to recommend the following:

- Eat raw foods whenever possible and without any seasoning.
- Use low temperatures to cook food.
- Steaming or oven cooking is healthier.
- Never burn foods.
- Boil water before cooking vegetables (boil vegetables for a short period of time as vitamins and minerals will remain in the water).
- Avoid reheating food once cooked.
- Consume first cold press olive oil.
- Never fry proteins (the oil that covers said proteins impedes the pepsin from our digestive tract to act on the proteins to be able to digest them).

- Add oil to food once it is already cooked.

BE SURE TO COMPLETELY COOK CERTAIN FOODS!!

It is very important to completely cook foods to kill any dangerous microorganisms that they may contain. Special attention should be paid to foods such as: ground beef, stuffed meats or roulade, large pieces of beef and chicken, fish, pork and eggs.

Regarding beef, chicken and fish:

These foods should be cooked until high temperatures are reached in their interior and until the juices are no longer pink. The inside as well as the outside of these foods contain a great amount of bacteria which makes it fundamental to cook them thoroughly throughout.

Eggs should be cooked until both the yolk and whites are completely done.

- HOW TO STORE FOOD

Raw foods, especially beef, chicken, fish and their juices, may contain dangerous microorganisms that can contaminate other foods during preparation and storage.

All raw foods should be stored separately from cooked foods, and old food should be stored away from fresh food to prevent the transfer of said microorganisms. Cooked foods may be contaminated by the smallest contact with raw foods or with a surface or utensil that has been in contact with raw foods.

Separate raw beef, chicken and fish from other foods when shopping for groceries to avoid the contamination of foods that will be eaten raw by their juices, such as certain vegetables or fruits.

Store food in covered recipients to avoid contact between raw and cooked foods.

Store cooked foods in the upper-most shelf and raw meats (deer, pork, chicken and/or fish in the lowest shelf to avoid any leakage of the juices onto already cooked foods.

Try to consume foods on the same day that you prepare them and try to cook only the quantity of food that you will be eating that day to avoid having any leftovers.

DON'T forget to separate fresh foods from old foods!!

Old foods can contain microorganisms that may contaminate fresh foods if they are mixed. Take advantage of old foods by eating them, if they are in proper conditions to be eaten, as soon as possible.

KEEP FOOD AT SAFE TEMPERATURES

Microorganisms quickly multiply if prepared foods are left more than 2 hours at room temperature and thus it is recommended that they be kept in the refrigerator soon after they are prepared. Food should be either very hot or very cold, given that microorganisms cannot reproduce in these conditions or can only do so very little. Therefore, store cooked foods and perishables – those that can go bad – at temperatures preferably below 40°F (5°C).

Don't keep your refrigerator too full as this makes it difficult for the cold air to circulate. Clean and thaw the refrigerator and freezer regularly.

DO NOT leave the refrigerator door open for long periods of time as this causes the temperature inside the refrigerator to change.

Foods can still rot when staying in the refrigerator or freezer. You should write the date when the food has been prepared on the recipient to know how long they can be kept.

Cool and store leftovers immediately. To avoid storing too many leftovers, **DO NOT** cook large amounts of food, but only what you think you will eat that day.

DO NOT store food for long periods of time, even if refrigerated. Consume any leftovers 2 or 3 days after preparation.

Pay attention to expiration dates and throw any expired foods away.

If you have frozen food, do not thaw at room temperature, but on the lowest shelf of your refrigerator.

- FOOD STORAGE TIME

Eggs: Raw in shell: 3-5 days; cooked: 1 week. Eggs must be kept at a temperature around 39°F (4°C) and they must be kept in their original carton packaging. Throw away any broken or cracked eggs.

Milk: 7 days in the refrigerator at around 39°F (4°C). Dairy products should be bought at the end of your shopping trip to keep them as cold as possible.

Butter: 1 to 3 months in the refrigerator at around 39°F (4°C). It must be well covered as it tends to absorb flavors from other foods.

Yogurt: 7 to 14 days in the refrigerator at around 39°F (4°C). Keep in its original packaging.

Sour cream: From 7 to 21 days, and once opened, use before 10 days.

Cheeses: Cheddar or Swiss, 6 months (unopened) in its original packaging to protect it from mold; brie, 3-4 weeks once open; grated, 1 week; fresh cheese or ricotta, 7-14 days. This type of cheese should be kept in its original packaging, stored upside down to preserve freshness, at around 39°F (4°C).

Meats: Ground meats, 1-2 days; quartered, 3-5 days; filleted, 3-5 days; stew leftovers, 3-4 days; grilled meat and meatballs, 1-2 days. All meats should be kept in the coldest part of the refrigerator, in the original packaging or in bags at around 39°F (4°C).

Poultry: Chicken or turkey, whole or quartered, 1-2 days at 39°F (4°C), stored in the coldest part of the refrigerator.

Fish: Low fat fish such as sole or cod, 1-2 days. Fatty fishes (salmon, halibut), 1-2 days. Cooked fish can be kept 3-4 days. All should be stored in the refrigerator at 39°F (4°C). To avoid odors, fish should be kept in airtight containers.

Shellfish: Shrimp, scallops, clams, mussels: 1-2 days. Live clams or lobster, 2-3 days. Cooked shellfish, 3-4 days. All should be stored at 39°F (4°C). Always wash your hands with soap and water after handling these products.

Fruit: Refrigerated: apples, 1-3 weeks; strawberries and raspberries, 1-2 days; citrus (orange, lemon, lime, etc.) and grapes, 5 days; fruit juices, 6 days and melons, 1 week. Room temperature: avocados, bananas, peaches, pears and apricots, 3-5 days. The latter ripen at room temperature. Once ripe, they are best stored in the refrigerator.

Vegetables:

Refrigerated: asparagus and green beans, 1-2 days; carrots and celery, 1-2 weeks; lettuce (romaine hearts), 3-5 days; lettuce (leaves or chopped), 1-2 days; mushrooms, 1-2 days; spinach, 5-7 days; corn on the cob, 1-2 days. All at 39°F (4°C). Asparagus should be kept in a vertical position in a recipient with 2-3 cm of water. Wash chopped lettuce leaves and stores them in an airtight container. Use absorbent paper towels to eliminate any excess humidity and keep them fresh.

At room temperature: onions, up to 4 weeks; potatoes, 2-3 months, and sweet potatoes, 2-3 weeks. Temperature: 44-50°F (7-10°C). Onions should be kept in a dry place; do not store them with potatoes as they produce humidity. They will last longer with a bit of circulating air. Tomatoes, 1-3 days. Tomatoes ripen at room temperature, away from direct sunlight.

Bread: Sliced, 5-7 days; French bread or baguette, 1 day. Rye or homemade bread, 2-3 days. Store bread loafs in the original packaging. Bread can be kept in the refrigerator so that it lasts longer, but it becomes stale and dry quickly.

Grains: Whole grains once packaging is opened, up to 2 months; grains unopened original packaging, up to 18 months and rolled oats up to 3 months. Use airtight containers to store grains or store grains in their original packaging for them to last longer. Rolled oats must be kept away from humidity and insects.

- FROZEN FOOD STORAGE TIME

Baked foods

Baked bread	12 months
Bread dough with yeast, unbaked	2 weeks
Breads with dried fruit or nuts	3 months
Rolls, unbaked	2 weeks
Baked rolls	12-15 months
Sweet rolls	3 months
Crepes, pancakes or waffles	6 months

Beef, pork, chicken and fish

Ground beef	3-4 months
Grilled beef	6-12 months
Beef fillets	6-12 months
Beef sausages/hot dogs	1- 2 months
Cooked beef dishes	2-3 months
Ground pork	3-4 months

Pork chops	4-6 months
Grilled pork	4-6 months
Pork sausage/hot dogs	1-2 months
Cooked ham	1-2 months
Stews/soups with ham	1-2 months
Bacon	1 month
Whole chicken (raw or cooked)	12 months
Quartered chicken (raw)	9 months
Quartered chicken (cooked)	4 months
Whole turkey (raw or cooked)	12 months
Stews/soups with poultry	2-3 months
Fresh (raw) fish (whole or quartered)	6 months
Cooked fish	3 months

Other

Cooked pasta	3-4 months
Cooked rice	3-4 months
Soups and stews (vegetable and/or meat)	2-3 months

1.1.4. ASSOCIATIONS

The rules regarding the association of foods are based on the knowledge that we have on the physiology of digestion and the chemical reactions that the nutrients found in food go through. We should take them into account in our dietary habits.

Above all, and without going into great scientific detail, I want to give you a brief explanation of the digestive apparatus so that you can understand how it functions.

The human digestive apparatus is composed of three cavities: the mouth, the stomach and the intestines. Each one secretes different digestive fluids to digest foods and we could thus say that digestion is carried out in three phases.

The nutrients contained in the foods we eat could not be absorbed and used by our bodies without digestion. Said nutrients must be reduced to the size necessary to pass through the intestinal walls and enter into the bloodstream.

Poor digestion favors fermentation and putrefaction that are the cause of many health problems. Understanding the actions of certain enzymes to comprehend the digestive process is very important.

Digestion starts in the mouth. The first enzyme that acts on foods is the alpha-amylase, which initiates the digestion of carbohydrates by reducing dextrin and maltose. In order for the amylase to continue its action, it needs an alkaline environment in the stomach. If no proteins are ingested, the gastric fluids secreted have a neutral pH. If the stomach secretes gastric fluids that are too acidic, the digestion of carbohydrates stops immediately.

Pepsin and gastric lipase are the enzymes found in the stomach. Pepsin acts on the digestion of proteins and requires an acidic environment to function. Lipase acts on fats, but an acidic environment inhibits the action of this enzyme.

When salivary and gastric digestion is carried out normally, the food is prepared for intestinal digestion where pancreatic enzymes and bile take action. The final products of hydrolysis are obtained in the intestines and the digested food will be prepared for absorption.

Intestinal secretions contain enzymes that need an alkaline environment to perform their functions. Some of them are shown below with a brief description of their action in the digestive process:

- **Enteropeptidase**: activates trypsin (the pancreatic enzyme that hydrolyzes protein molecules by converting them into smaller peptides).

- **Erepsin**: completes the function carried out by the pepsin and trypsin, hydrolyzing peptides to obtain amino acids.

- **Maltase**: acts on the maltose and dextrin, products of the salivary digestion of starches.

- **Sucrase**: hydrolyzes sucrose to obtain glucose and fructose.

- **Lactase**: hydrolyzes lactose, the sugar found in milk.

Bile, secreted by the liver and poured into the duodenum, performs many important functions in the small intestine. It can be considered as a coenzyme of the pancreatic lipase. When combined with bile, it decomposes fats quickly and favors the absorption of fatty acids by making them more soluble. It also helps in the assimilation of many fat-soluble vitamins, such as vitamin D, E and K.

After having briefly explained digestion, I will now talk about the association of foods by explaining the action of each food association with its consequences.

1.1.3.1. FERMENTATION, PUTREFACTION AND CONSEQUENCES

Many physiologists defend the fact that fermentation and putrefaction are normal phenomena that are constant and necessary for digestion and nutrition.

Accepting simple common observations as normal is outrageous.

We know today that bacteria from putrefaction reduce proteins to amino acids and destroy them, creating the following toxins as a final product: indole, skatole, phenol, acids, carbon dioxide, hydrogen, hydrogen sulfide, ammonia, alcohol, etc.

All of these toxins perturb and destroy intestinal flora leaving the intestines permeable, which allows for them to pass into the bloodstream.

And blood? Where does blood circulate? Through absolutely all of our organs and other parts of our organism (bones, joints, muscles, skin, genitals, glands, brain...) From this, a broad range of symptoms arise whose origin are, in most cases, a mystery that conventional medicine cannot solve.

Regardless, due to the accumulation of gasses in the abdomen, the bad breath produced by gastrointestinal fermentation and putrefaction, the fetid and unpleasant odor of feces and gasses that are expelled, are as undesirable as the poisons that produce them.

The blood stream should receive water, amino acids, fatty acids, glycerol, monosaccharides, minerals and vitamins, and never alcohol, acids or ammonia.

We must clearly understand that we can preserve good breath, not produce gasses and have odorless feces. We can free our body from the burden of having to oxidize and eliminate toxins.

The digestion of foods by enzymes makes them usable by the human body, while their decomposition by certain bacteria makes them useless and unusable for the organism's needs. The first process produces nutritional elements as a final product, and the second produces poisons.

In short, in order to nourish ourselves, the foods that we ingest must be digested and not rot in the process.

We must ask ourselves what are the causes of fermentation and putrefaction in the digestive tract. They may be due to overeating, erroneous combinations of foods, the use of condiments, lemon, vinegar, eating under emotional or physical conditions that delay or suspend digestion (fatigue, excessive work, concerns, fear, anxiety, pain…), etc.

Millions of euros are spent yearly on drugs that only achieve the temporary relief of these discomforts. Chemical substances to neutralize acids, to reabsorb fats or alleviate pain are used massively by many people. Other substances, such as pepsin, are used in disproportionate quantities as an aid to facilitate digestion.

All of these phenomena are extremely abnormal. Tranquility and well being, and the lack of pain and discomfort, are signs of good health. Any signs or symptoms of illness do not accompany normal digestion.

1.1.4.2. ACID-BASE BALANCE (PH)

The idea of the acid-base balance is fundamental and is part of daily life hygiene. But what do "acid" and "base" or "alkaline" mean? What is "pH" or a "buffer system"?

pH is a unit of measurement of the degree of acidity or alkalinity of a liquid. Its value is measured using a scale that goes from 0 to 14:

- From 0 to 7 is acid
- 7 is neutral
- From 7 to 14 is alkaline.

Biological liquids that have a pH under 7 are called acid solutions and those with a pH over 7 are called base or alkaline solutions. Blood, for example, has a slightly alkaline pH of 7.4 (considered as stable between 7.36 and 7.42). Each organ functions optimally in a specific acid-base environment. Optimal pH oscillates from 6.4 and 6.9 (6.5 – 7.0).

These values have a greater importance in the proper functioning of vital processes. Indeed, in a live biological system, any large and abrupt variation of pH values may endanger survival. There are protective systems to avoid abrupt or large variation of pH, called "buffer systems". These are found throughout our entire organism.

When the acid-base balance of an organ is broken it means that the conditions of the pH were not respected. Therefore, said organ will not function optimally and its digestive process will be disturbed. pH imbalance causes the following metabolic problems, among others:

- Imbalance of the metabolism of carbohydrates: obesity or diabetes;
- Imbalance of sodium: retention of liquids;
- Imbalance of proteins: rheumatism or renal problems;

Below we see what can cause this imbalance and the possible consequences or effects on our health.

- CAUSES OF ACID-BASE IMBALANCE

- Excessive overload of acids from eating: a diet low in fresh foods, excessive ingestion of proteins, refined foods or saturated fats.

- Formation of acids and other toxins produced by fermentation.

- Shortage of vitamins, trace elements, and minerals.

- Fatigue.

- Chronic stress.

- Physical stress.

- Lack of oxygenation of tissues.

- Chronic kidney failure: failure in the elimination of toxins by skin and kidneys.

- Endocrine pathology: diabetes…

- Intoxication by heavy metals.

- EFFECTS OF ACID-BASE IMBALANCES

Demineralization: that simultaneously causes irritation of skin and mucous membranes and, therefore, lowers defenses against microorganisms.

Suppression of the immune system: that may lead to the formation of mineral deposits, that is, stones of all types (bladder, kidney, gall, salivary) and joint sclerosis.

Symptoms:

- Chronic fatigue.

- Tiredness and feelings of being cold.

- Difficulties in recovering from illness or injuries.

- Tendency towards depression.

- Swollen and sensitive gums.

- Sensitive teeth (to cold, hot or acidity).

- Cavities.

- Dull hair.

- Dry, cracked skin.

- Fragile, scratched or spotted finger and toenails.

- Rectal burning sensation

- Cramping or muscle spasms.

- Joint pain.

- High receptivity to infections.

- TREATMENT OF ACID-BASE IMBALANCE

My philosophy in this aspect is "treatment". The best treatment is prevention, with proper hydration and a varied and balanced diet.

On this basis, my dietary recommendations are the following:

- Diets should be less acid and more alkaline;
- The primary source of alkaline substances are from foods, basically all fruits and vegetables;
- Minerals are important for the acidifying or alkalizing behavior of foods;
- Drink two liters of mineral water per day;
- Eat enough proteins, vitamin D and get enough

oxygenation…

A great indicator: URINE

The kidneys eliminate excess acids. A simple and precise way to verify what is occurring in our organism is through our urine.

The system to verify this value is very simple: a pH indicating strip. These paper strips are impregnated in a substance that changes color when in contact with acid or base substances. When compared to a scale, we know, with good precision, the pH of the substance in question, in this case, urine.

A healthy and well-balanced person that receives enough alkaline substances in their diet will present a slightly alkaline pH in the second urination in the morning, identical to the pH of blood.

The first urination in the morning cannot be used, as it is naturally acid. Nocturnal rest allows kidneys to eliminate acid product waste.

- LIST OF ACIDIFYING FOODS

FATS AND OILS

Avocado oil
Corn oil
Flaxseed oil
Lard
Olive oil
Safflower oil
Sesame oil
Sunflower oil

FRUITS

Blueberries

NUTS AND BUTTERS

Cashews
Brazil nuts
Peanuts
Peanut butter
Pecans

ANIMAL PROTEINS

Beef
Carp
Clams
Fish
Lamb
Lobster

MEDICATIONS AND CHEMICALS

Chemical medications
Medicinal medications
Psychedelics
Pesticides
Herbicides

ALCOHOL

Beer
Spirits
Hard liquor
Wine

BEANS AND

GRAINS

Rice cakes
Amaranth wheat cakes
Barley
Buckwheat
Corn
Oats
Quinoa
Rice (all types)
Rye
Spelt
Kamut
Wheat

DAIRY PRODUCTS

Cow's milk cheese
Goat's cheese
Processed cheese
Sheep's cheese
Milk
Butter

Mussels
Oysters
Pork
Rabbit
Salmon
Shrimp
Tuna
Turkey
Deer

PASTA (WHITE)

Noodles
Macaroni
Spaghetti

OTHER

Distilled vinegar
Wheat germ
Potatoes

LEGUMBRES

Black beans
Garbanzos
Peas
Broad beans
Lentils
Pinto beans
Red beans
Soy beans
Soy milk
White beans
Rice milk
Almond milk

- LIST OF ALKALIZING FOODS

VEGETABLES

Garlic
Asparagus
Fermented vegetables
Watercress
Sugar beets
Broccoli
Brussels sprouts
Cabbage
Carrots
Cauliflower
Celery
Swiss chard

FRUITS

Apple
Avocado
Banana (high glycemic index)
Melon
Cherries
Currant berries
Dates/figs
Grapes
Grapefruit
Lime
Honeydew melon

OTHER

Apple cider vinegar
Bee pollen
Soy lecithin granules
Probiotic cultures
Green juices
Vegetable juices
Fresh fruit juices
Mineral water
Antioxidant alkaline water
Green tea
Herbal tea
Dandelion tea

Chlorella
Leafy greens
Cucumber
Eggplant
Kale
Lettuce
Mushrooms
Spicy leafy greens
Sweet leafy greens
Dandelions
Edible flowers
Onions
Peppers
Squash
Sea plants
Spirulina
Sprouts
Pumpkin
Alfalfa
Barley grass
Wheat grass
Wild leafy greens
Purple lettuce

Valencia melon
Nectarine
Orange
Lemon
Peach
Pear
Pineapple
All berries
Mandarin orange
Tropical fruits
Watermelon

PROTEIN

Eggs
Chicken breast
Vegetal yogurt
Almonds
Chestnuts
Tofu (fermented)
Flaxseeds
Pumpkin seeds
Tempeh (fermented)
Squash seeds
Sunflower seeds
Millet seeds
Walnuts

Ginseng tea

SWEETENERS

Stevia

SPICES/CONDIMENTS

Cinnamon
Curry
Ginger
Mustard
Powdered chili
Sea salt
Miso
Tamari
All herbs

ASIAN VEGETABLES

Maitake mushroom
Dailon
Dandelion root
Shitake mushroom
Kombu (kelp)
Reishi mushroom
Nori (seaweed)
Umeboshi
Wakame
Sea vegetables

1.1.4.3. FOOD GROUPS

Below, I provide you with a simple classification of the foods that constitute the base of our nutrition, grouped according to properties and possible mixtures based on their composition, that is, their primary nutrients (proteins, carbohydrates, fats, vitamins, minerals and trace elements).

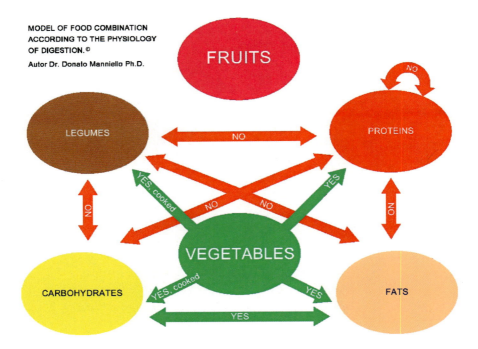

GROUP 1: VEGETABLES

These are foods that lack animal proteins, with a low amount of carbohydrates, which provide us with fiber, vitamins and minerals.

They can be combined with any type of food.

Lettuce	Leek	Endive
Cabbage	Pepperns	Rocket
Mushrooms	Cucumber	Lamb's lettuce
Broccoli	Turnip	Watercress
Chard	Eggplant	Sprouts
Spinach	Green beans	Dandelion
Garlic	Celery	Radish
Onion	Asparagus	Rhubarb
Squash	Belgian Endive	Chicory

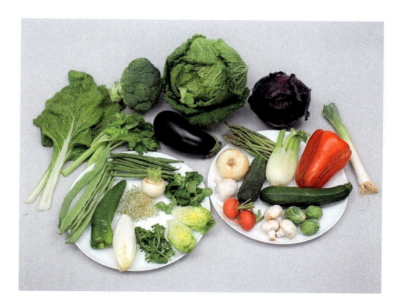

GROUP 2: CARBOHYDRATES

This group includes starches, sugars, etc.… In short, carbohydrates, both with short and long chains, whose principal function is to provide energy.

They can be mixed with other carbohydrates. Mixing more than two types is not recommended. They can be associated with cooked vegetables and fats.

Grains (wheat, millet, oats, spelt, rye, quinoa, soy, couscous…).

Whole wheat bread	pastas	rice
Pumpkin	potato	Carrot
Artichokes	cauliflower	yam
Salsify	corn	beets

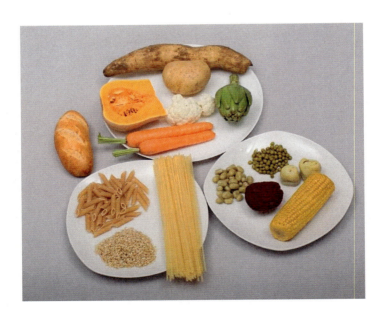

GROUP 3: LEGUMES

Legumes are complex foods that have a similar proportion of carbohydrates and proteins and, therefore, are difficult to classify in either of these two groups. They should be associated with cooked vegetables.

- Lentils
- Dried beans
- Black beans
- Red beans
- Chickpeas
- Peas
- Broad beans

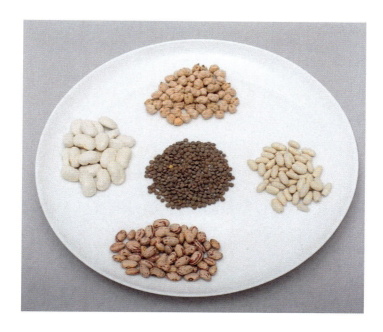

GROUP 4: PROTEINS

All foods that possess a high percentage of proteins from animals are included in this group.

Different types of proteins cannot be mixed among themselves

(Meat and fish, meats and eggs, fish and eggs…)

You can mix fishes between them.

Meats can be mixed with other meats.

They can be associated with raw or cooked vegetables.
Beef, pork, lamb, chicken, turkey, fish, seafood, etc…
Eggs.
Tofu.

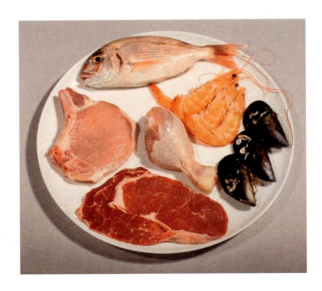

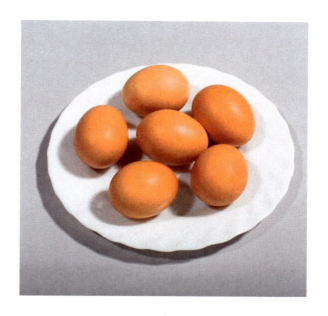

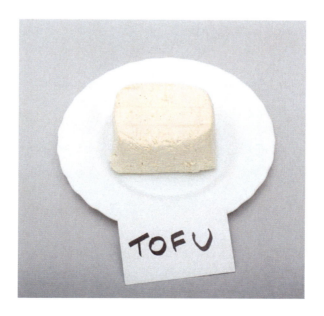

GROUP 5: FATS

Foods that are principally or solely composed by lipids of the fatty acid type belong to this group.

There are many types of fats and oils. I list below some of the healthiest options.

Extra virgin olive oil.
Sesame, almond, walnut, sunflower and flaxseed oils…
Avocados.
Olives.
Soy butter.

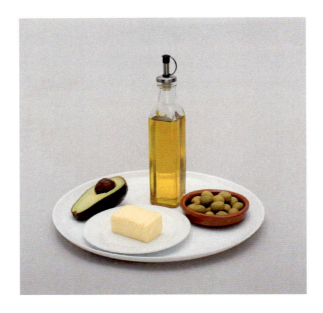

GROUP 6: FRUITS

Fruits are divided into neutral, sweet, semi-acidic and sour. Mixing any fruit from one group with a fruit from another group is not recommended, neutral oils fruit and sweet sugars, ferments to produce toxic cellular life. Nor are compatible with acidic, because acid when mixed with sugars, they retard the formation of glucose, staying longer than normal in the intestines, which produces toxic fermentations. When mixed, could cause certain symptoms in the body such as headaches, nausea, stomach discomfort, indigestion, acidity, and even diarrhea. All fruit should be eaten away from meals.

NEUTRAL FRUIT: (can be eaten morning or afternoon)

Avocado	Chestnuts	Peanuts
Almonds	Walnuts	Hazelnuts
Coconut	Corozo fruit	Cocoa
Macadamia nuts		

SWEET FRUIT: (can be eaten morning or afternoon)

Apricot	Plum (various types)	Mangosteen
Dragon fruit	Sugar Apples	Dates
Apples (various types)	Watermelon	Banana
Pomegranate	Melon	Grape (various types)
Currant	Loquat (various types)	Zapote
Cayman	Soursop	Papaya
Cherry	Guava (various types)	Papayuela
Cherimoya	Fig	Pear

SEMI-ACID FRUITS: (can be eaten in the morning)

Caimito	Strawberry	Green Apple
Plum (various types)	Granadilla	Marañón
Jocote	Guava	Quince Meat
Lime	Loquat (various types)	Peach
Physalis	Peach	Tangerine
Raspberry	Mango	

ACID FRUITS: (can be eaten in the morning)

Cranberry	Lemon	Pineapple
Grape	Borojo	Apple (various types)
Piñuela	Cayman	Passion Fruit
Grapefruit	Blackberry	Tamarind
Kiwi	Orange	Tomato

Some recommendations for the consumption of fruits:

- Wash fruits thoroughly
- Preferably eat organic fruit
- Do not combine fruits with vegetables at the same time
- Do not combine fruits from different fruit groups
- Preferably eat acidic fruits late morning
- Eat sweet fruits anytime
- Fruits should be eaten fresh and ripe
- Do not drink fruit juices during or after meal times
- Some fruits should be eaten or drunk alone: Orange, Pineapple, Melon, and Watermelon

* This list could grow with further research.

1.1.4.4. INCORRECT ASSOCIATIONS

- ASSOCIATION: CARBOHYDRATES AND PROTEINS

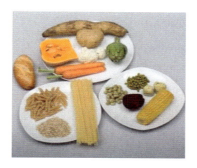

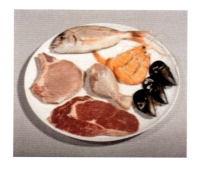
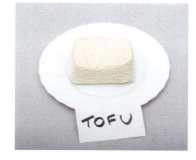
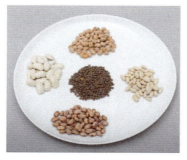
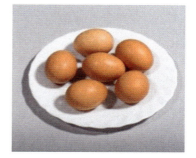

Meats with potatoes, fish or chicken with rice, pasta with Bolognese sauce, Spanish omelet (omelet with potatoes), rice with eggs, etc.

Salivary digestion, or the action of the amylase on carbohydrates, takes place as you chew your food until it reaches the stomach and needs and alkaline medium. Starches are not completely digested until they reach the small intestine, where their hydrolysis is continued. If they spend too much time in the stomach, it is likely that they begin to ferment and decompose, due to the adequate temperature of this organ for said phenomena.

If we eat proteins at the same time that we eat carbohydrates, the stomach secretes pepsin with acidic secretions due to the presence of the proteins that immediately cancels out the action of the amylase. This process quickly paralyzes the digestion of starches and they will begin to ferment.

Fermented starch will quickly coat the pepsin and it will thus lose its action on proteins. This means that neither the carbohydrates nor the proteins will be digested for at least two hours. Digestion is then carried out through fermentation and as a result we will suffer from abdominal bloating, gasses, etc. In short, you will feel heavy and sleepy.

- ASSOCIATION: CARBOHYDRATES AND ACIDS

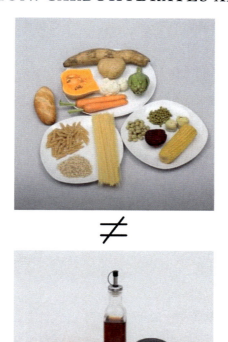

When we ingest acids (acidic fruits, tomato, vinegar, lemon, certain medications, etc.), the action of the amylase is detained and carbohydrates cannot be digested. It will later be reduced in the small intestine by pancreatic enzymes.

This is why I recommend not eating carbohydrates and acids in the same meal.

- ASSOCIATION: CARBOHYDRATES AND RAW VEGETABLES

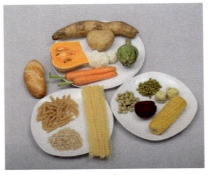

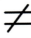

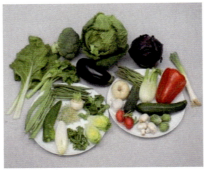

Summer salads, tabouleh, rice, pasta or potato salads with raw vegetables, bread or toast with raw tomato...

All of this seems healthy, right? Vegetables are not digested in the stomach, but later in the duodenum and the rest of the small intestines.

What really happens is that the association makes the carbohydrates retain the raw vegetables in the stomach, causing fermentation, with all of the respective disadvantages that we already know about.

- ASSOCIATION: CARBOHYDRATES AND SUGARS

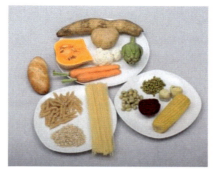

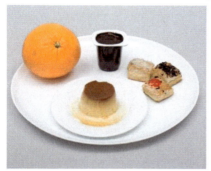 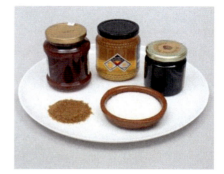

Jams, compotes, sweet fruits, honey, molasses, syrups, sugar (white and brown)…

As you already know, sugars are only digested in the small intestine. We also know that when we place something sugary in our mouths, we salivate and the liberation of myalase is scarce or non-existent. In this case, the carbohydrate ingested with said sugar will not be digested.

When we associate sugars with carbohydrates, the later pass slowly through the stomach, impeding their digestion, and they quickly cause an acidic fermentation.

- ASSOCIATION: PROTEINS AND PROTEINS

Meats, legumes, eggs,...

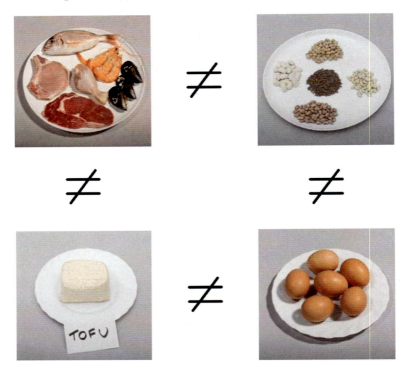

We know today that each protein needs time and different digestive conditions according to its specific characteristics. For example, eggs receive a more concentrated secretion at a different time than meat.

The digestive process is different and is modified for the digestion of each type of protein. It is impossible for the organism to cater to two different types of proteins in the same meal. The final result is the fermentation of one of the proteins.

At the same time, different types of meat, cheese or nuts can be associated. However, the following associations should be avoided: meat and eggs, meat and legumes, meat and fish, eggs and legumes...,

- ASSOCIATION: PROTEINS AND ACIDS

Acidic fruits, raw tomato, vinegar, lemon, acidic substances used in salad dressings...

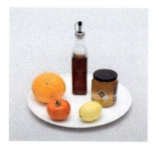

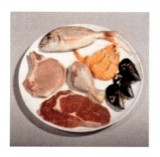

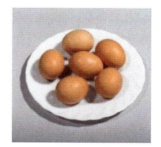

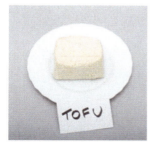

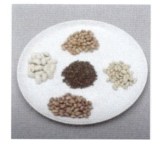

We know that pepsin is the enzyme that digests proteins. We also know that pepsin is activated and functions in an acidic medium and only in the presence of hydrochloric acid. But if the medium is very acidic, the pepsin will be destroyed and the proteins will not be digested, activating the process of putrefaction of said proteins.

Errors are sometimes committed: some people believe that adding acids to their foods will help digestion. The presence of some kind of acid in the mouth or in the stomach will impede the activation of gastric acids and the liberation of pepsin.

Following this rule, we should never associate proteins with acids in the same meal.

- ASSOCIATION: PROTEINS AND FATS

Frying meats, accompanying with cream, butter, all types of oil, sauces…

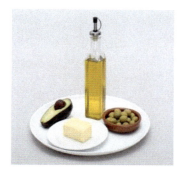

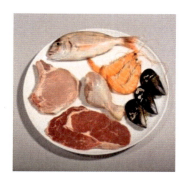
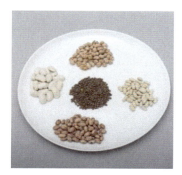
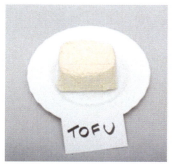
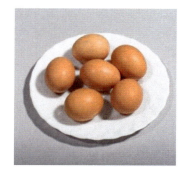

It has been shown that the presence of fats in foods reduces the volume of the secretion of gastric fluids, hydrochloric acid and the amount of pepsin. This inhibitory effect may last two or more hours. The ingestion of abundant green vegetables at meals counteracts the inhibitory effect of fats.

- ASSOCIATION: PROTEINS AND SUGARS

Dairy desserts, ice-cream, fruit, honey, pastries, etc.... after eating meat, eggs or legumes...

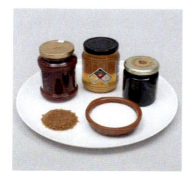 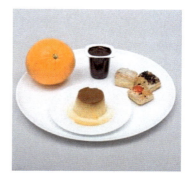

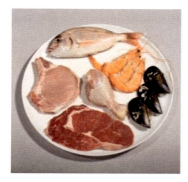 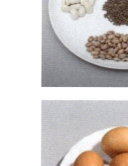

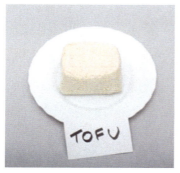

We know that sugars are not digested in the mouth or the stomach, but in the intestines. If they are eaten alone, they do not stay in the stomach very long and they pass quickly through the intestines. When they are associated with proteins, they stay in the stomach, which impedes their digestion and favors, once again, fermentation.

Also, the "sweet" effect activates the opening of the pylorus (a valve that controls the passage from the stomach to the small intestine) that allows for the proteins to pass, having yet to be digested, to the duodenum. We know that the duodenum and the small intestine are not able to digest proteins and this then ferment and putrefaction takes place.

Dumping gastric syndrome or rapid gastric emptying is a syndrome in which ingested food leaves the stomach quickly and goes largely into the small intestine without being digested. This syndrome occurs when the upper end of the small intestine, the duodenum, expands too quickly due to the presence of hyperosmolar foods in the stomach.

In addition, people with this syndrome often suffer from hypoglycemia because rapid expulsion of food causes the pancreas to release excessive amounts of insulin into the blood. This type of hypoglycemia is known as "reaction hypoglycemia"

- SUMMARY

AVOID:

- RAW FRUITS AND/OR VEGETABLES WITH CARBOHYDRATES (bread, pasta, rice, potatoes. For example, typical summer salads).
- CARBOHYDRATES AND PROTEINS (meats, chicken, fish…).
- ASSOCIATING ALL 3: CARBOHYDRATES, RAW VEGETABLES AND PROTEINS.
- DRINKING WATER DURING MEALS (which hinders digestion).

- FRUIT AND SWEET DESSERTS AFTER MEALS.
- MIXING SWEET FRUIT WITH ACIDIC FRUIT.
- EATING LARGE AMOUNTS IN THE MORNING (the stomach later asks for similar large amounts throughout the day).

YOU CAN:

- PROTEINS WITH RAW OR COOKED VEGETABLES.
- CARBOHYDRATES WITH COOKED VEGETABLES.
- FRUIT AND WATER (2 liters/day) ONLY BETWEEN MEALS.
- ONLY HAVE ONE PLATE OF FOOD AND CHEW THOROUGHLY.
- ONLY EAT FOODS THAT YOU TOLERATE WELL (if possible, don't try those that cause intolerances).

GENERAL DAILY PROPORTION

60% VEGETABLES AND FRUIT

20% WHOLE GRAINS AND CARBOHYDRATES

20% PROTEINS (1g of protein/kilogram of weight/day)

Note: 100 gr of beef, fish or chicken = +/- 20 gr of protein.

1.1.4.5. CORRECT NUTRITIONAL HEALTH GUIDELINES FOR ONE WEEK

It is clear that the balanced ingestion of foods will be done according to needs and taking into account age, sex, life style, exercise habits, etc.

Your diet should be varied, rotational and you should eat five times per day.

Set a stable schedule for your meals.

Rest after lunch. There is a Spanish saying that says "Rest after lunch and walk after dinner".

Dinner should be eaten three hours before going to bed.

Remember to chew your food thoroughly before swallowing.

Consume an abundant amount of fruit, vegetables, whole grains and legumes.

Eat nuts and dried fruits.

Moderate the consumption of salt, sugar and alcoholic beverages.

Decrease the total consumption of fat, saturated fat and cholesterol.

SUMMARY OF THE FOOD GROUPS

GROUP 1: VEGETABLES

These can be mixed among themselves.
They can be combined with all types of food.

Lettuce	Leek	Belgian Endive
Cabbage	Pepper	Endive
Mushrooms	Cucumber	Lamb's lettuce
Broccoli	Turnip	Watercress
Chard	Eggplant	Sprouts
Spinach	Green beans	Dandelion
Garlic	Celery	Radish
Onion	Asparagus	Rhubarb
Squash	Cardoon	Chicory

GROUP 2: CARBOHYDRATES

These can be mixed among themselves and mixing more than two is not recommended.

These can be associated with cooked vegetables and fats.

Cereals (wheat, millet, oats, spelled, rye, quinoa, soy, couscous ...)

Whole wheat bread	Pasta	Rice
Pumpkin	Potatoes	Carrot
Artichokes	Cauliflower	Yam
Salsifies	Corn	Beets

GROUP 3: LEGUMES

Only associate with cooked vegetables.

Lentils
Dry beans

Black beans
Red beans
Chickpeas
Peas
Broad beans

GROUP 4: PROTEINS

These cannot be mixed among themselves (meat and fish, meat and egg…).
The different meats can be mixed among themselves.
The different fishes can be mixed among themselves.
Raw or cooked vegetables can be associated with the proteins.

Beef, pork, lamb, chicken, turkey, fish, shellfish, seafood
Eggs.
Tofu.

GROUP 5: FATS

These can be associated with vegetables and carbohydrates.

Extra virgin olive oil.
Sesame, almond, walnut, sunflower and flaxseed oils…
Avocados, olives, soy butter.

"Graves are full from large dinners"
(Spanish saying)

"Let food be your nutrition and your nutrition your medicine"
(Hippocrates)

BREAKFAST

Coffee or tea + with/without plant-based milk + whole grain cookies w/o wheat.

OR only fruit.

OR fruit + soy yogurt.

OR soy yogurt + sugar-free whole grain cereal.

OR oat/soy/rye/rice drink + cereal.

OR WHEAT-FREE whole grain bread with olive oil + herbal tea.

MID-MORNING

Fruit (acidic fruits only in the morning, sweet fruits in the morning/afternoon).

Or 1 soy yogurt + herbal tea.

Or fruit smoothie

LUNCH

3 days per week eat: group 1 + 2 + herbal tea.

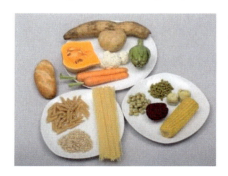
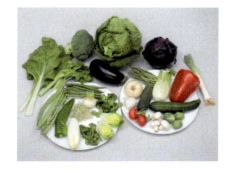

2 days per week eat: group 1 + 3 + herbal tea.

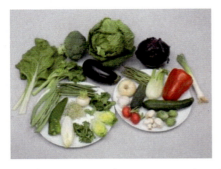 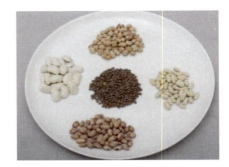

2 days per week eat: group 1 + 4 + herbal tea.

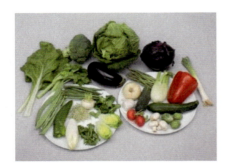 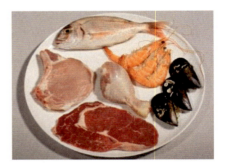

You can choose whatever you want from each group and associate it with whatever else you want from the other group!

Example:

MONDAY	group 1+2
TUESDAY	group 1+3
WEDNESDAY	group 1+4
THURSDAY	group 1+2
FRIDAY	group 1+3
SATURDAY	group 1+4
SUNDAY	group 1+2

AFTERNOON

Sweet or neutral fruit

Or 1 soy yogurt + herbal tea.

Or fruit or vegetable smoothie

DINNER

Each day eat: group 1 + 4 + herbal tea.

Except the days that you eat proteins at lunch: eat group 1 + 2

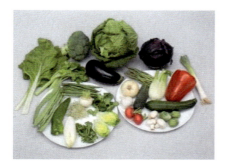
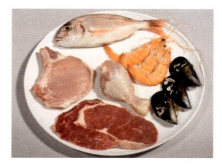
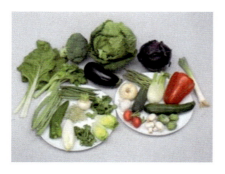
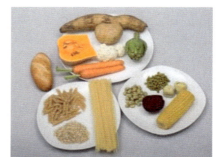

THE APPLICATION THAT WILL CHANGE YOUR LIFE

With the Manniello Method App you will be able to:

. Create personalized healthy menus for a whole month.

. Recommendations to eat healthier.

. Recommendations to combine and cook food.

. Automatic shopping list.

Why choosing Manniello Method App?

Compared to other mobile applications, this one presents an innovative dietary method based upon more than 25 years research and proven on more than 4000 patients. Amounts and calories are not imposed!

What can it offer you in your daily life?

Improve your life quality by rebalancing your organism functions. Improvements are noticeable between 10 days and a month: better digestion, weight loss and balance, sleep and mood improvement...

What does it imply in your overall health?

Sickness recovery, Immune system boost, vitality and vigour... to help you achieve your objectives.

Do you want to improve your health and lifestyle?

Download the app in:

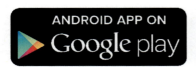 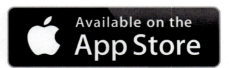

MANNIELLO METHOD RECIPES

- RICE WITH RATATOUILLE +/- 20 min.

. In a saucepan lightly fry a clove of garlic with a spoonful of extra virgin olive oil. Add 100 gr of rice and let it fry for a minute. Cover it with twice its volume of water and add a pinch of salt. Cover the pan and let it cook over low heat.

. Chop all the vegetables into cubes. In a pan fry an onion and aubergine with olive oil. Then add 1 zucchini/courgette and 1 red pepper. Then add 1 tomato, salt, pepper, 2 bay leaves. Cook over low heat.

- NOODLES WITH BROCCOLI AND MUSHROOMS +/- 15 min.

. In a saucepan of water and a pinch of salt cook 200gr of noodles al dente.

. In a pan fry 1/2 broccoli and 6 mushrooms chopped with 2 cloves of garlic and 4 tablespoons of extra virgin olive oil. Once the noodles are cooked, strain them and add them to the broccoli and mushrooms. Mix together and serve.

- BAKED POTATOES WITH VEGETABLES +/- 25 min.

. Cut up and place on a baking tray 4 potatoes, 1 red onion, 1 zucchini/courgette, 1 red pepper, 2 artichoke hearts, 1 sprig of thyme, 1 sprig of rosemary, extra virgin olive oil, salt, and bake.

- SAUTE OF CHICKEN WITH VEGETABLES +/- 15 min.

. Chop and slowly sauté a chicken breast, with a little lemon and salt.

Add (sliced) ½ zucchini/courgette, ½ onion, 1 red pepper, 1 green pepper, salt and spices to your liking.

- GRIDDLED STEAK WITH SALAD +/- 15 min.

. Cook the meat in a pan without oil, always over low heat, add organic salt at the end of cooking. Accompany with a sauce made with garlic, parsley and salt. Add rocket or lamb's lettuce.

- BAKED FISH WITH 3 PEPPERS +/- 20 min.

. Cook 2 fillets of hake or other white fish, salt, pepper and aromatic herbs.

. In a pan sauté the red, green and yellow peppers with extra virgin olive oil and a clove of garlic, salt.

- LENTILS WITH AUBERGINE AND ZUCCHINI/COURGETTE +/- 25 min.

. Soak 200 g of lentils overnight in a bowl of water. Sauté a clove of garlic with extra virgin olive oil and add the lentils. Then cover them with twice their volume of water. Add a spring onion stuck with with 3 cloves. Then add 1 sliced aubergine and 1 sliced zucchini/courgette, salt and 2 bay leaves. Cook over low heat.

- CHICKPEAS WITH SPINACH +/- 25 min.

. Soak 200 gr of chickpeas overnight in a bowl of water. Sauté a chopped onion in extra virgin olive oil and add the chickpeas. Then cover them with twice their volume of water. Then add 300 gr of fresh spinach, salt and 2 bay leaves. Cook over low heat.

- WHITE BEANS WITH CHARD AND PEPPERS +/- 25 min.

. Soak 200gr of white beans overnight in a bowl of water. Sauté a chopped onion in extra virgin olive oil and add the white beans. Then cover them with twice their volume of water. Then add 300gr of chopped chard, 1 red pepper and 1 green pepper, salt and spices. Cook over low heat.

- TOMATO SAUCE 1

. In a saucepan sauté a clove of garlic in a spoonful of extra virgin olive oil. Add 6 chopped plum tomatoes, 6 basil leaves, salt. Cook over low heat.

- TOMATO SAUCE 2

. In a saucepan, sauté a chopped onion in a spoonful of extra virgin olive oil. Add 6 chopped plum tomatoes, ½ chopped red pepper, salt and 2 bay leaves. Cook over low heat.

- TOMATO 3 SAUCE (FOR PIZZAS)

. In a saucepan sauté 2 finely chopped cloves of garlic in 1 tablespoon of extra virgin olive oil. Add 400 ml of tomato puree, salt and 2 tablespoons of oregano. Cook over low heat.

- VEGAN MAYONNAISE (To accompany your baked potatoes)

. In a glass, a little wider and taller than the blender, put

1 glass of sunflower oil

1/3 glass of soy or oat milk

1/2 clove of garlic

Salt

Beat at low speed. Once the mixture has blended at the bottom, move the mixer little by little, so that it blends the oil that is on the surface of the mixture.

- BECHAMEL SAUCE (To accompany your vegetables, rice or potatoes)

. 50 gr buckwheat or white oat flour

50 gr Soy margarine

500 ml Vegetable milk (soy, oat)

Nutmeg

Salt

Melt margarine in a saucepan, taking care not to burn, because it would give the whole dish a bitter taste. Over low-medium heat, add the flour, little by little, stirring constantly to make a smooth paste. Turn it over a few times so that the flour browns slightly. Then add the milk little by little, and again stir it so that everything blends well together. Let the dough cook over medium heat for a while, so that the flour is not raw. Adjust the salt, and add a little freshly grated nutmeg.

- PESTO (to accompany your pasta)

2 cups fresh basil (gently pressed)

1/2 cup of pine nuts (other options are walnuts or almonds)

1 or 2 cloves of crushed garlic

1/2 cup extra virgin olive oil

Salt and pepper to taste

Put the basil, pine nuts and garlic in the blender (we can also do it with the mortar and pestle). Beat to a thick paste. Then add the olive oil little by little while continuing to grind the mixture. Salt, pepper. Grind everything together a little more until you get the right texture.

MOJO VERDE (To accompany your meat or fish)

1 head of garlic (8-10 cloves)

1 bunch of coriander

1 teaspoon of cumin seeds

15 tablespoons of olive oil

1 teaspoon of salt

Beat all the ingredients with the blender adjusting the consistency with a little water.

- CHIMICHURRI (To accompany your meat or fish)

- 1 head of garlic (8-10 cloves)

- 1 bunch of parsley

- One teaspoon of paprika (sweet or spicy)

- 1 teaspoon of cumin seeds

- 15 tablespoons of olive oil

- 1 teaspoon salt

Beat all the ingredients with the blender, adjusting the consistency with a little water.

- MUSHROOM OMELETTE

. Sauté 200 gr of assorted mushrooms with a clove of garlic and extra virgin olive oil, fresh parsley, salt and pepper to taste. Beat 2 eggs with a pinch of salt and add to the mushrooms, cover the pan and cook over low heat. Serve accompanied by young salad leaves.

- OMELETTE WITH 3 PEPPERS

. Sauté 200 gr of red, green and yellow peppers with half a chopped onion and extra virgin olive oil, fresh chives, salt and pepper to taste. Beat 2 eggs with a pinch of salt and add to the peppers, cover the pan and simmer. Serve accompanied by lamb's lettuce and rocket.

- OMELETTE WITH ZUCCHINI/COURGETTE

. Sauté 200 gr of zucchinI/courgette with half a chopped onion and extra virgin olive oil, fresh coriander, salt and pepper to taste. Beat 2 eggs with a pinch of salt and add to the zucchini/courgette, cover the pan and simmer. Serve accompanied by sprouted grains.

- MACARONI WITH EGGPLANT/AUBERGINE AND ZUCCHINI/COURGETTE

. Sauté in extra virgin olive oil half an aubergine and half a zucchini/courgette cut into cubes with half a chopped onion, half a diced tomato, 5 green olives (stoned), salt, and turmeric to taste. Cook the macaroni al dente. Mix the macaroni with the vegetables for a moment so that the flavours are blended.

- MUSHROOM RISOTTO

. Prepare 1 liter of vegetable stock (750 ml of water with 2 vegetable stock cubes). Sauté 200 gr of assorted mushrooms and a clove of garlic in extra virgin olive oil, salt. In a saucepan sauté a clove of garlic and add 150 gr of rice, over low heat. Add a ladle of broth to the rice and keep stirring. Add the broth until the rice is cooked and creamy. 5 minutes before finishing add the mushrooms, fresh parsley and grated soy cheese.

- STEWED RIBS WITH VEGETABLES

. Sauté half a chopped onion in extra virgin olive oil with half an aubergine, half a zucchini/courgette cut into cubes, 10 chopped flat beans, a red pepper, salt and cumin to taste. Cover with double the volume of hot water and add 10 meaty pork ribs. Cook over low heat until the ribs are done. (+/- 25 minutes)

- CURRY STEW CHICKEN WITH VEGETABLES

. Sauté half a chopped onion with extra virgin olive oil, broccoli, 5 mushrooms, half a zucchini/courgette cut into cubes, 10 pea pods, a chopped red pepper, salt and curry to taste. Cover with twice the volume of hot water and add 10 pieces of chicken. Cook over low heat (+/- 25 minutes)

- VEGETARIAN PIZZA GLUTEN FREE

. Buy the gluten-free pizza base in a supermarket. Add a layer of tomato sauce for pizzas (see recipe), then add slices of aubergines, zucchini/courgette, mushrooms, red pepper, artichokes, corn, salt, (optional: vegetable cheese). 20 minutes in the oven (180°) Serve with extra virgin olive oil and chopped basil.

- PIZZA WITH MUSHROOMS AND BLACK OLIVES GLUTEN FREE

. Buy the gluten-free pizza base in a supermarket. Add a layer of tomato sauce for pizzas (see recipe), then add assorted mushrooms, black olives, vegetable cheese. 20 minutes in the oven (180°) Serve with truffle oil.

- PIZZA WITH ONIONS WITHOUT GLUTEN

. Buy the gluten-free pizza base in a supermarket. Sauté with extra virgin olive oil over low heat 3 sliced onions, salt. Place the onions on the pizza, oregano (optional: vegetable cheese as a base). 20 minutes in the oven (180°)

SMOOTHIES, FRUIT JUICES AND VEGETABLE JUICES

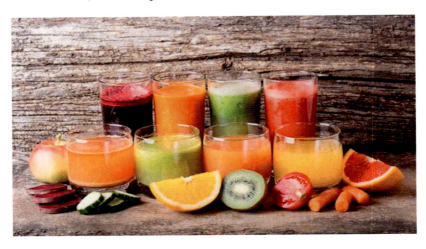

We all know how important and essential vitamins and minerals are for health.

These nutrients are bioavailable in fruits and vegetables. Every day the body needs these "fuels" for the cells and metabolism to work properly.

A very simple way to provide them is in the form of juices or smoothies. The only difference is that the juice is made with an extractor obtaining the liquid without the fibers so that it is bioavailable directly in the intestines avoiding all the work of digestion. The smoothy is simply fruits or vegetables with 200 gr of crushed ice beaten in the blender for 3 minutes.

These juices and smoothies can be taken alone at breakfast, mid-morning or as an afternoon snack. The benefits are numerous: they

- balance the metabolism

- regulate weight

- assuage hunger pangs

- balance the hormonal system

- detoxify the organism

- reduce body fat

- reduce inflammation

- balance blood sugar

-tone your energy ...

In this way you will steer your organism towards alkalinity, nourishing, remineralizing, hydrating and detoxifying yourself.

All the recipes are prepared according to their therapeutic effect and they are made easily (as juice alone with the extractor or as a smoothie with 200 gr of crushed ice beaten in the blender for 3 minutes) They take between 10 and 15 minutes to prepare and are for 2 servings.

Important information: Fruits are divided into neutral, sweet, semi-acidic and acidic. Remember that you should not mix any fruit of one group with fruit of another group. If they were mixed, it would cause a fermentation in our body, which could cause certain symptoms such as headaches, nausea, stomach pain and others.

There are even fruits of the same group that should not be combined, such as orange, melon, watermelon and pineapple. These fruits should be consumed alone.

You cannot mix fruits and vegetables because they have a different digestion time in the intestine and that would also cause fermentation.

The Manniello Method respects the correct combinations of foods to avoid all fermentation in the body. Always wash all foods thoroughly with water and baking soda before use.

DETOXING AND DEPURATIVE RECIPES

With fruits

1. . 200 gr of grapes

    . 2 apples

    . 2 Pears

2. . ½ papaya

    . 3 apples

    . 100 ml of water

3. . 200 gr of plums

    . 2 pomegranates

    . 100 gr of cherries

4. . 400 gr of watermelon

    . 1 cup of mint herbal infusion

5. . ½ melon

    . 1 cup of white tea

6. . 200 gr of strawberries

    . 3 peaches

    . 100 ml of water

7. . 4 pink grapefruit

    . 1 lemon

    . 2 kiwis

8. . ½ pineapple

   . 1 cup of green tea

With vegetables (It can be seasoned with cayenne pepper, berries, nutmeg ...)

1. . 4 sticks of celery

   . 100 gr of parsley

   . 100 gr of watercress

   . 200 gr pumpkin

   . 1 cucumber

ANTIOXIDANT RECIPES

With fruits

1. . 200 gr of grapes

   . 2 apples

   . 100 gr of cherries

2. . 100 gr of raspberries

   . 200 gr of strawberries

   . 1 mango

3. . 100 gr of plums

   . 2 peaches

   . 4 tangerines

4. . 100 gr of blueberries

. 1 lemon

. 2 grapefruit

. 1 kiwi

With vegetables (They can be seasoned with cayenne pepper, berries, nutmeg ...)

1. . 300 gr of chards

    . 200 gr of spinach

    . 300 gr of carrots

2. . 300 gr of kale

    . 200 gr of chard

    . 300 g of pumpkin

3. . 300 gr of kale

    . 200 gr of spinach

    . 300 gr of sweet potato

4. . 4 sticks of celery

    . 2 cucumbers

    . 2 tablespoons fresh coriander

    . 2 tablespoons fresh parsley

    . 1 beetroot

SLIMMING RECIPES

With fruits

1. . 4 apples

    . 2 peaches

    . 1 cup of green tea

2. . 200 gr blackberries

    . 200 gr blueberries

    . 3 pink grapefruit

With vegetables

(It can be seasoned with cayenne pepper, berries, nutmeg ...)

1. . 400 gr of spinach

    . 3 cucumbers

    . 1 red pepper

    . 1 clove garlic

ENERGIZING RECIPE

With fruits

. 3 pink grapefruit

. 1 lemon

. 3 green apples

. 1 piece of ginger

2. PHYSICAL HEALTH: DAILY EXERCISE

"Exercise is the most effective method held by medical science to preserve, conserve and recover the health of human beings depending on the specific case of each individual".

(Cristóbal Méndez – 1555)

2.1. INTRODUCTION

Currently, it seems to be clearly demonstrated that while a sedentary lifestyle is a factor of risk to develop numerous chronic diseases, among which cardiovascular diseases stand out as they represent one of the principal causes of death in the western world. A physically active lifestyle produces many benefits, both physical and psychological, for good health.

According to the WHO (World Health Organization), health can be defined as "the complete state of physical, mental and social well being and not only the absence of diseases".

One of the reasons to exercise is to search for the state of wellbeing that approaches the individual concept of health as a basic component of quality of life.

2.2. BENEFITS OF PHYSICAL ACTIVITY

According to research, it seems that there is a relationship between physical activity and life expectancy. More active populations tend to live longer than less active populations.

Likewise, people who regularly exercise have the subjective sensation of feeling better than they did when they did not exercise, from both physical and mental perspectives, that is, they have a better quality of life. It seems clear, therefore, that exercising has a positive impact on health.

The human body has been designed to move and it requires regular exercise to stay functional and avoid getting sick. Physical activity is any body movement produced by muscles and that requires spending energy.

Physical exercise is a type of physical activity that is defined as "all programed, structured and repetitive body movement performed to improve and maintain one or more of the components of being in shape". A sedentary lifestyle is when the level of physical activity does not reach the minimum needed to maintain a healthy state.

According to statistics, 40 to 60% of the population has a sedentary lifestyle, and only one of every five individuals reach the minimum physical activity recommended for good health.

"Physical exercise is the method to live more years in your life and more life in your years"

(Dr. K. H. Cooper)

There currently seems to be enough evidence that proves that those people that live a physically active life experience a long list of health benefits. The following are some examples:

- Prevention of many diseases caused or aggravated by excess body weight: cancer, diabetes and cardiovascular diseases, among others.

- Improved function of internal organs, which in turn improves body functions such as breathing, digestion, elimination, etc.
- Stable blood pressure.
- Reduced cholesterol.
- Increased use of body fat and improved weight control.
- Aid in establishing cardio-healthy habits for life in children and fighting against certain factors (obesity, hypertension, hypercholesterolemia, etc.) that favor the development of cardiovascular diseases as adults.
- Improved mood and prevention against depression.
- Fortified bones and stronger muscles.
- Aid in maintaining joint structure and function.
- Decreased risk of falls in elderly people, aid in delaying or preventing chronic diseases and those that are associated with aging.
- Increased body energy.
- Increased secretion of hormones that increase the vitality of humans and their wellbeing.
- Increased sexual health.
- Improved sleeping patterns.
- Stress control.
- Increased oxygenation of the brain, which improves mental

performance.

- Increased skin appearance and health as sweating favors a process of detoxification by activating circulation and effectively slows down the aging process.

However, and in spite of all the previously mentioned benefits, anyone who plans on starting an intense physical activity program that has any kind of chronic disease (ischemic heart disease, arterial hypertension, diabetes, etc.) or a high risk of having them, and for women over 50 years of age and males over 40, should have a physical examination beforehand.

2.3. WAKING UP IN THE MORNING

The awareness of movement is important for a healthy lifestyle with which we work to maintain our body and mind as healthy and vital as possible. Movement should be manifested as a natural manner of living, as education and as the promotion of good health.

According to traditional Chinese medicine, and the theory of the four times, the exteriorization of energy starts at six o'clock in the morning. This is when everything starts to move, we come out of deep sleep, we slowly open our eyes and we begin to stretch.

Before getting out of bed, carrying out a few stretches is recommended to help wake our physical body. Try the following:

Lay down on your back, with a pillow under your neck. Start making circles in one direction and then the other, with your feet and hands, for one minute.

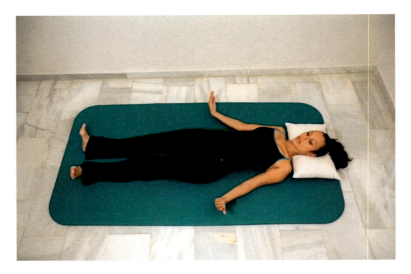

In the same position, flex your elbows bringing your hands to your shoulders ten times.

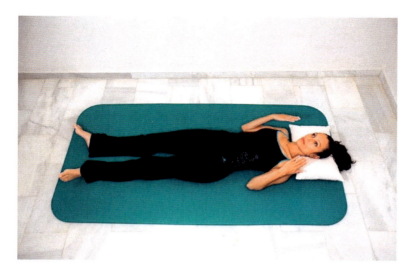

In the same position, lift your arms to a vertical position (reaching to the ceiling) ten times.

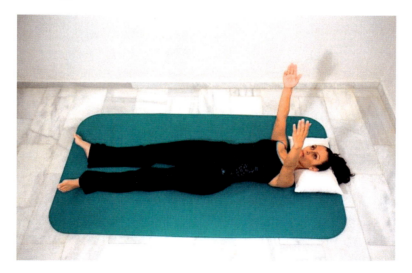

In the same position, lift your arms to a horizontal position (like a snow angel) ten times.

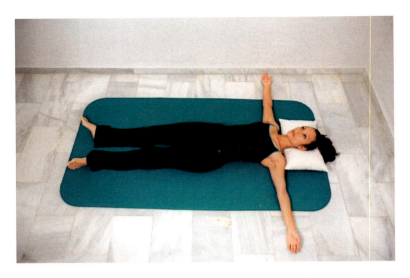

In the same position, move your head smoothly ten times to the right and left.

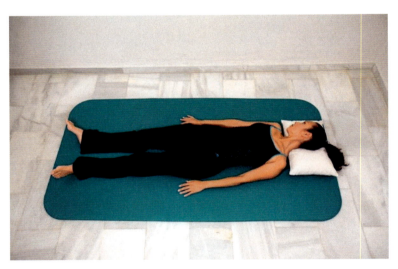

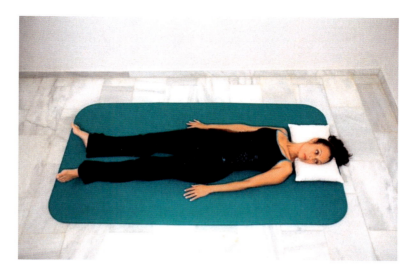

In the same position, incline your head smoothly ten times to the right and left.

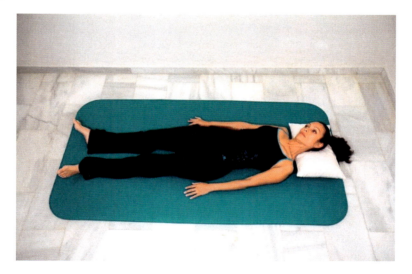

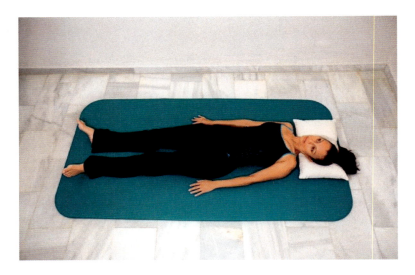

Bend your knees with your feet flat on the bed. Pull your knees into your chest with your arms straight. Lift your head toward your knees and hold the position for ten seconds and then relax keeping your knees in your hands. Repeat five times.

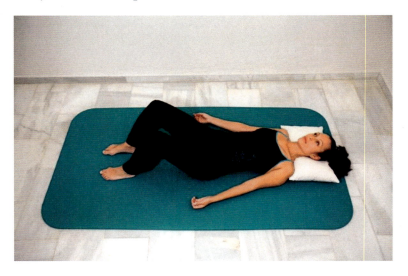

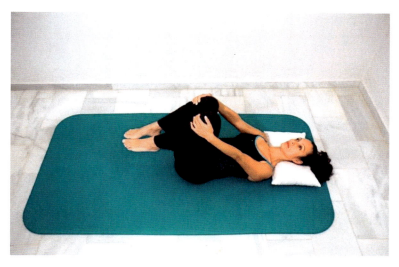

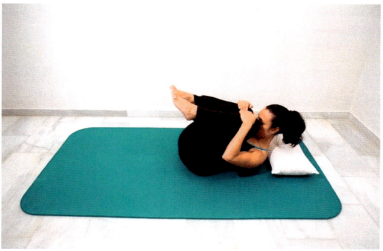

In the same position, cross one leg over the other. Hold the knee that is underneath with both hands. Pull that knee towards your chest and hold for ten seconds. Relax, keeping your knee in your hands. Repeat five times.

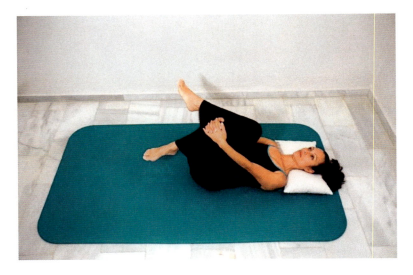

Do the same movement with the other knee.

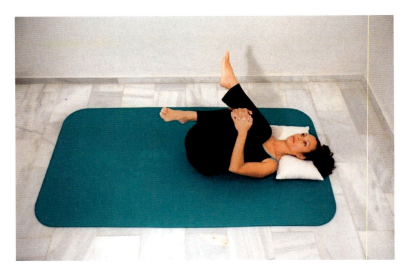

In this same position, with your feet on the bed, place your left foot over your right leg. With your left hand, push the left knee down. Hold the pose for ten seconds and then relax. Repeat five times.

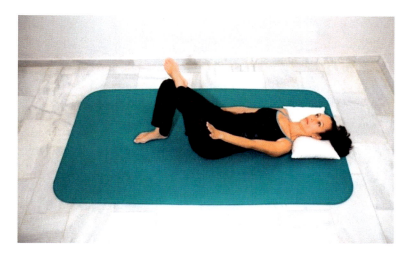

Do the same movement with the right foot.

In the same position, with your arms open, bring your knees to your chest. In this posture, move your bent knees to the right side without changing the position of your arms. Hold the position for ten seconds while looking in the other direction. Do the same for the left side. Repeat twice.

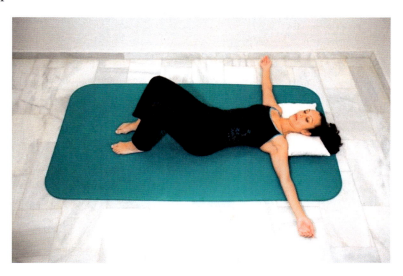

TAKE ME WITH YOU AND I WILL CHANGE YOUR LIFE

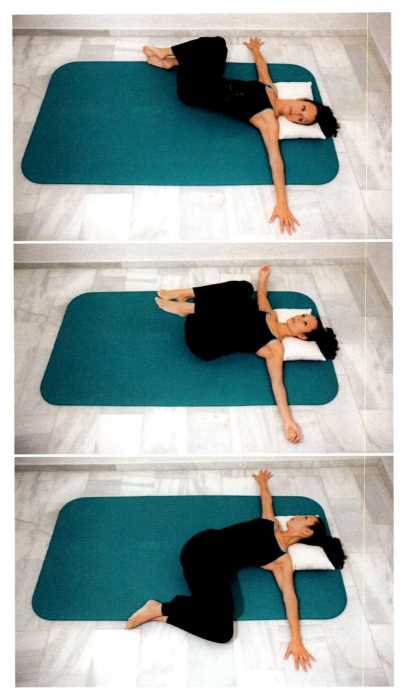

Your body is now ready to get up and have breakfast. At the same time, how we get out of bed is also important:

-First, lay on your side;

-Bend your knees and move your legs out of the bed for balance;

-Place one hand close to the other elbow and push yourself up.

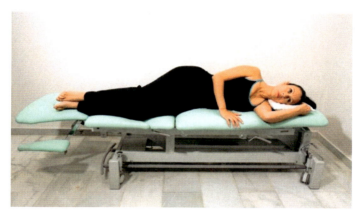

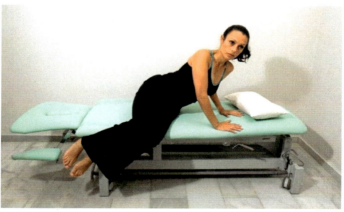

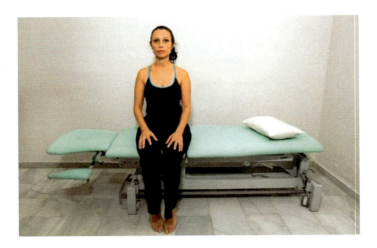

Yoga, qi cong or tai chi can also be used to start your day in a healthy manner that will wake you up and fortify your energy.

2.4. WALKING 30 MINUTES A DAY

"Is there anything easier, cheaper and healthier?"

Many people spend hours at the gym, sweating, and sometimes overdoing it and harming their bodies. What is the need for this? Is it a passing fashion?

Without looking down on the benefits that certain people gain from exercising at these centers, I recommend a much simpler, less tiring, free form of exercise that is available for people of all ages…I'm talking about walking, clear and simple.

Walking is the most effective benefit for many of our health problems. It is a physical activity that benefits us in all aspects, both mentally and physically.

Walking requires no special complements (clothing, devices, etc.) like other sports do, although wearing proper footwear that cushions and protects your feet is recommended.

A few of the many benefits of walking include:

- Improved sleeping patterns and reduced signs of depression.
- Decreased risk of suffering from diseases related with the heart and diabetes.
- Fights obesity and improves blood circulation.
- Increases bone density, counteracting the effects of osteoporosis.
- Strengthens the muscles and tendons of legs and feet.
- Reduces the amount of harmful cholesterol in blood and stabilizes arterial blood pressure.
- Decreases anxiety and stress, increases the amount of

endorphins in the brain and creates a positive mental state and attitude.

- 120.   Raises self-esteem and encourages thinking.
- Stabilizes the spine.
- And, it also burns calories!

Walking should be done at a fast pace that makes us sweat and increase our heart beat slightly. According to research, walking is healthier than running as it does not strain joints in an excessive manner. To fortify the benefits of walking, it take deep breaths as you go. For example: breathe in for three steps and breathe out for the next three steps.

2.5. STAYING IN SHAPE

Minimally, the following exercises or going to the gym two or three times a week is recommended. Regular and adequate exercise is something that we should do daily.

2.5.1. STRETCHING

Stretching the different muscle groups before and after any physical activity is fundamental. Stretching prepares muscles for exercise. Stretches are done to warm-up and cool-down to avoid injuries. Also, periarticular muscles (those that cross a minimum of two joints, such as the biceps and quadriceps) perform better when they are more stretched out, physiologically speaking. Stretching should never be painful. If it is, lower the intensity until it does not hurt.

Follow the guidelines below to stretch the most important muscle groups.

Calf stretches: Standing up, with one leg forward and flexed, and the other one behind and straight. Move the heel of the straight (back) leg towards the ground until you feel the calf stretch. Hold for ten seconds, return slowly to the initial position and repeat three times, changing legs.

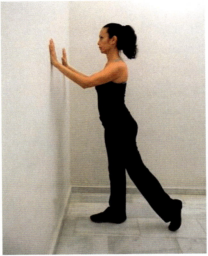

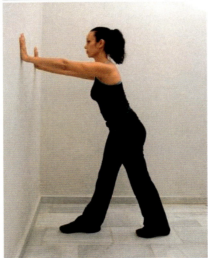

Quadriceps stretches: With one arm leaning on a wall, bend one leg bringing the foot toward your bottom, holding on with the hand of the same side. Hold for ten seconds, return slowly to the initial position and repeat three times, changing legs.

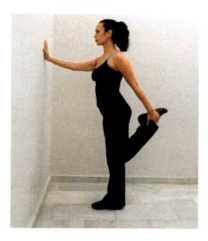

Hamstring stretches: Standing up, bend your trunk forward and down while keeping your legs straight. Hold for ten seconds, return slowly to the initial position and repeat three times.

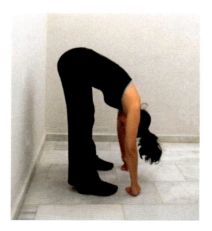

Sitting, with your legs straight out in front of you with your toes pointing straight up, bed your trunk forward towards your feet. Hold for ten seconds, return slowly to the initial position and repeat three times.

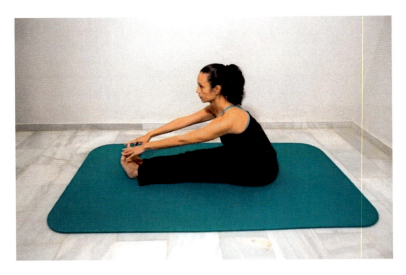

Biceps and forearm flexor stretches: Stretch your arm, with your palm facing upwards. With the other hand, flex the first hand down while keeping the elbow straight. Hold for ten seconds, return slowly to the initial position and repeat three times, changing arms.

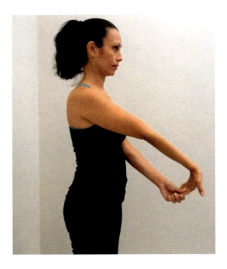

Triceps and dorso-lateral muscles: Place your hand towards the base of your neck. With the other hand, hold your elbow and pull towards the opposite side. Hold for ten seconds, return slowly to the initial position and repeat three times, changing arms.

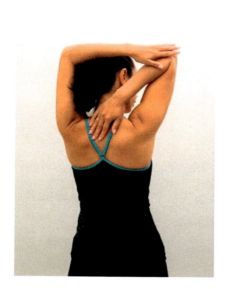 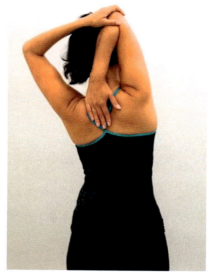

Pectoral stretches: standing up, elevate your elbows to a horizontal position with your hands on your collar bones. Stretch your elbows back two times then open your arms horizontally and stretch back again two times. Repeat ten times.

TAKE ME WITH YOU AND I WILL CHANGE YOUR LIFE

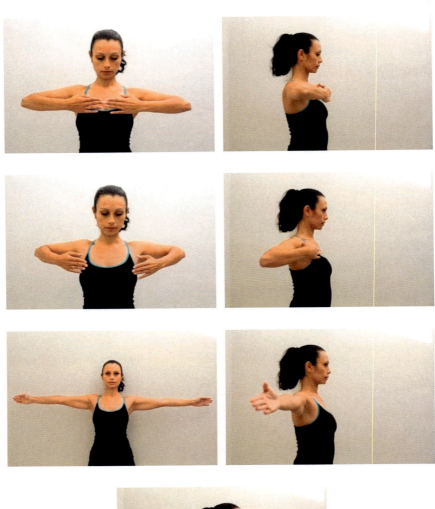

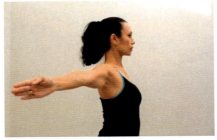

Trapezius stretches: Standing or sitting, let your head fall forward. With your right hand placed on the posterior left part of your head, gently stretch your head down diagonally to the right until you can feel the stretch in your trapezium. Hold for ten seconds, let go of your head slowly and return to the initial position. Repeat three times on each side.

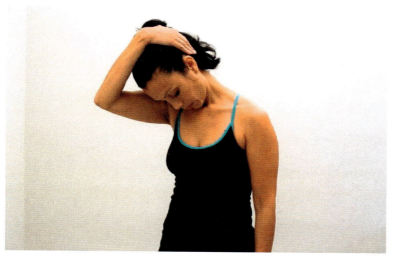

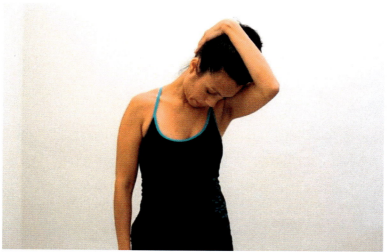

Lower back stretches: Lay down face-up, with your legs bent and your feet flat on the floor. Grab your knees with your hands and your arms straight. Pull your knees towards your chest and lift your head towards your knees. Hold the stretch for ten seconds and then relax while keeping your knees in your hands. Repeat five times.

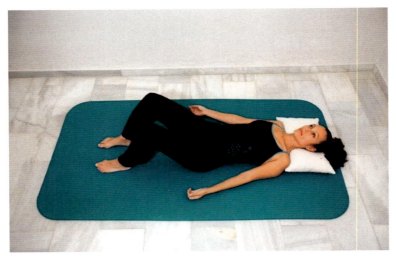

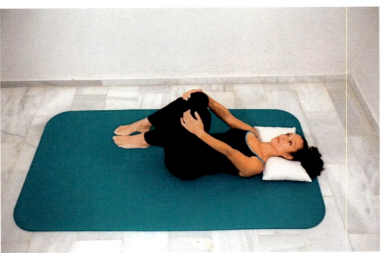

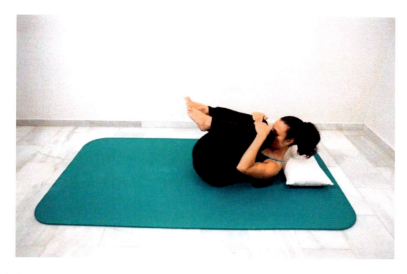

2.5.2. MAINTENANCE EXERCISES

Below I have listed a series of exercises that will help to keep you in shape. Exercise should always be appropriate for your age and physical condition, gradually increasing resistance and strength (you can add weights of half kilo, one kilo and up to two kilos to your wrists and ankles), and always with stretching and warm-up before and stretching and cool-down afterwards to avoid injuries.

Exercises for calves, quadriceps and hamstrings. Standing up, with your feet slightly apart, raise your heels and flex your knees to 130º. Hold the position for ten seconds, straighten your knees and lower your heels. Repeat ten times.

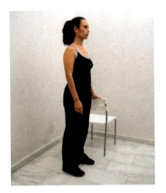
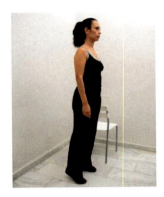
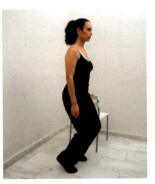
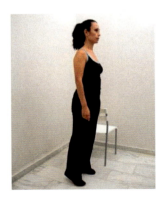
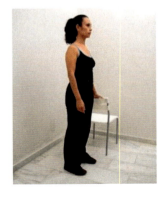

Exercises for abductors and adductors: Standing up and using a chair for support, lift your leg laterally to 45° while keeping your trunk straight. Hold the position for ten seconds and slowly return to the initial position. Repeat ten times with each leg.

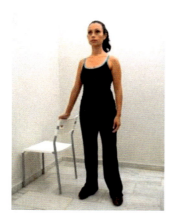
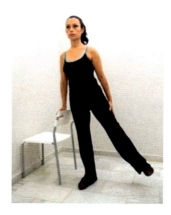

Exercises for gluteus: Standing up and using a chair for support, lift your leg back to 45° while keeping your trunk straight. Hold the position for ten seconds and slowly return to the initial position. Repeat ten times with each leg.

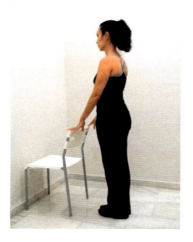
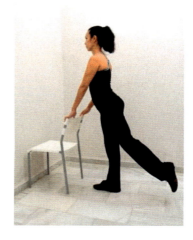

Exercises for pectorals, biceps, triceps and forearm flexors

and extensors: On all fours, with your arms in a vertical position and your shoulders aligned with your hands, flex your arms and move your chin towards the ground between your two hands. Repeat three series of ten.

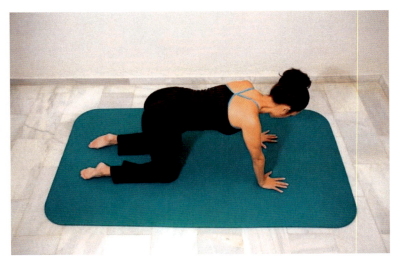

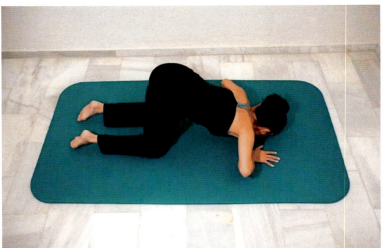

In the same position, repeat the same exercise but moving your chin to 20 cm in front of your hands.

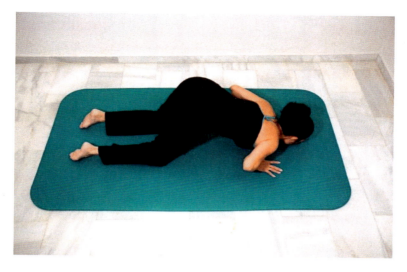

If the previous position is too easy, you can opt for the horizontal position supporting yourself with your hands and your feet (push-ups).

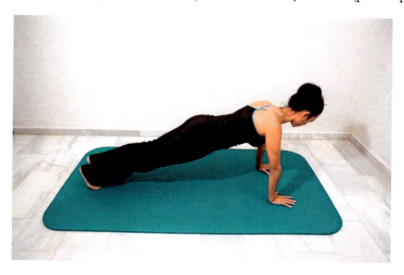

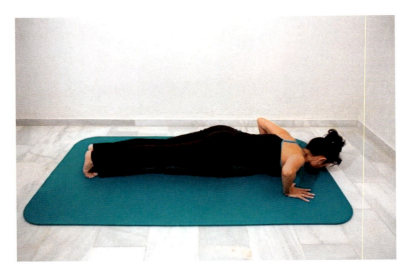

Exercises for the dorsal and interscapular muscles: Laying face down (placing a pillow below your stomach makes this exercise more comfortable), with your arms extended horizontally forward, with your neck straight (chin down), lift your arms no more than one centimeter. Hold the posture for five seconds and relax. Repeat ten times.

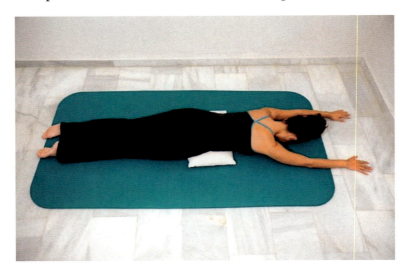

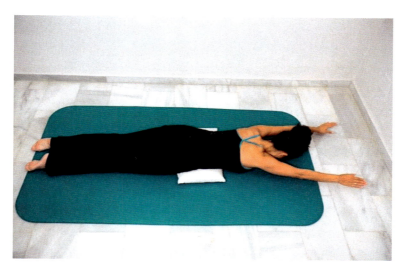

In the same position, with your arms stretched out laterally, with your palms facing down and your neck straight (chin down), lift your head no more than one centimeter and move your arms five times up and down and relax. Repeat ten times.

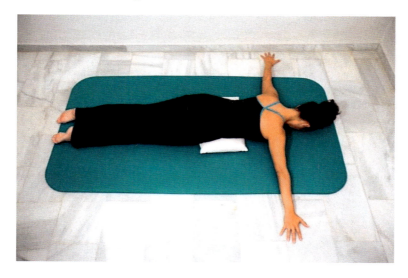

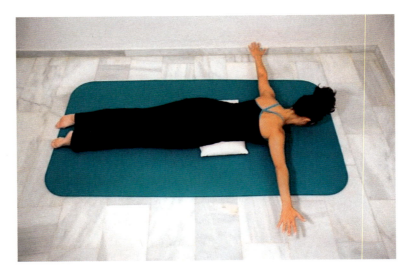

Exercises for the abs and obliques: lying face up, with your knees flexed and your feet flat on the floor, with your hands on your thighs, slide your hands until you touch your knees, lifting your head, neck and chest, and return to the initial position. Do three series of ten movements.

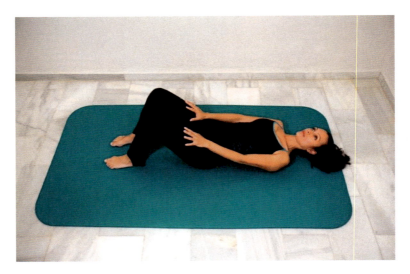

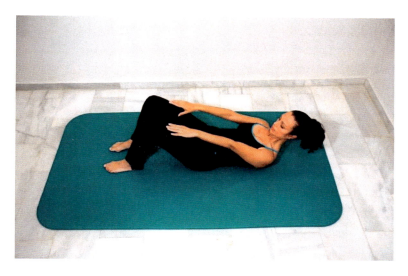

In the same position, but with one hand over the other, slide you hands towards the outer part of one of your legs and return to the initial position. Repeat towards the other side. Do three series of ten movements.

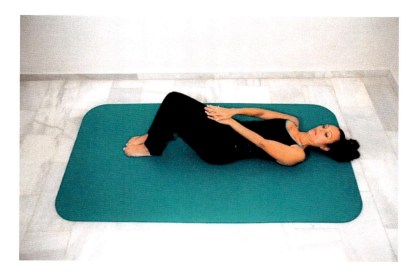

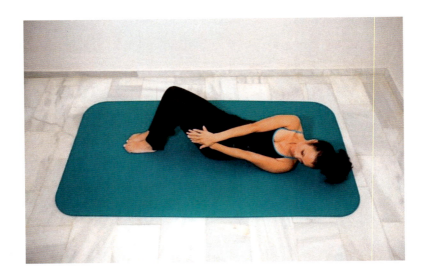

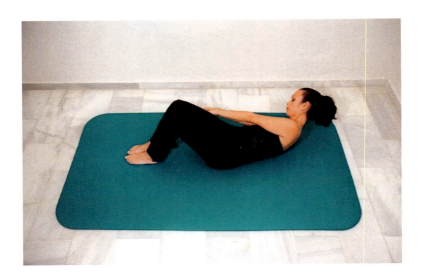

2.6. GOOD POSTURE HABITS

"The body is the instrument through which we manifest ourselves in this life. It is the vehicle that we use on the path of life. Taking care of it and keeping it in perfect conditions is our responsibility; regular exercise and good posture are fundamental"

(Dr. Gaspar García)

We spend most of our life sitting, laying down or in postures that harm the integrity of our spine. The lack of exercise, a result of a sedentary lifestyle, causes muscular weakness, especially of the muscles that protect the vertebral spine (abdominal, intervertebral, lumbar, trapezoids, dorsal).

A recent survey reveals that a huge percentage of the population suffers from or has suffered in the past from back pain (lower back and neck pain), and it is the first cause of missing work.

Adopting good postural habits would avoid these problems. I recommend the following:

- Always sit down to get dressed or undressed: socks, underwear, pants, shoes with laces...
- Flex your knees to pick something up from the floor.
- Keep your back straight when you are standing, sitting or walking.
- When carrying something, distribute the weight evenly between both arms.
- Never associate a flexion movement with a rotation movement at the same time.
- If you sleep on your side, your pillow should be firm and keep

your head in line with your spine.
- If you sleep face up, the pillow should keep your neck in a horizontal position.
- Avoid wearing high heel and platform shoes.
- When you work for a prolonged period of time in front of a computer screen, us a Swiss chair (a kneeling chair). This way, the spine adopts a correct posture in a natural way centered over your pelvis and the trapezoids are not overworked, which, in turn, strains the neck.

3. MENTAL HEALTH: THE POSITIVE MIND

"Luck does not exist in life, it is a logical sequence of events".

3.1. RESEARCH FINDINGS

There is a time in life when we realize that there is an abysm that exists between our deep aspirations and our daily life. It is an event that is lived and experienced in a painful manner, that we have rejected, which allows us to access this comprehension. Each one of us is a prisoner of a set of beliefs that makes us have inhibitory or reactive behaviors. This is what we call "memories from educational or social hypnosis".

We then feel trapped by routine and the habits of stressful daily activities, which seem artificial, lacking of coherence and authenticity. This is due to the fact that we protect ourselves from certain aspects of life that deeply disturb us.

These inhibitory or reactive behaviors, to face certain events, as a consequence of the non-spoken and non-done, impede us from expressing ourselves about this dimension of the heart that we feel behind these concerns.

This leads us to not knowing how to talk to each other, how to touch ourselves, how to be spontaneous…

We then ask ourselves: Who are we really? Why does life confront us with certain situations? Why do we suffer?

These existential-type questions, which are fundamental for a true awakening of our conscience, can find answers to liberate us of alienating memories, of emotional dilemmas that we carry around with us. We cannot become adults without becoming aware of and starting to rid ourselves of our shells, which restrain us from being, in the sense of freedom in action and thought.

3.2. THE TEACHINGS OF LIFE

Each one of our lives has a purpose and a meaning. All that we live from the moment of our conception forms a part of life's lessons. And each day, we learn a new lesson.

The goal of all we learn is to evolve in our worldly experience. This is only one stage, and it is not forever. This is why it is important that during this journey, our learning is as rich as possible. It is true that in some circumstances, this is not what happens. Due to the fact that we are all connected with everything, any thing can affect us. Our emotions determine how we perceive the environment that surrounds us.

When faced with any situation or event, we have two possible forms to react:

- sit down and cry in a corner asking ourselves: "Why me, why me?" (victim position);

- or we can ask ourselves: "What is life trying to show me with this lesson?" (spiritual evaluation position).

We have the capacity to decide how to allow life to affect us, to be as we wish to be, to feel as we wish to feel, to be or not to be happy...

"Happiness is hidden in the waiting room for happiness"

(Eduard Punset)

In the hypothalamus of the human brain, the "search circuit" is found. This circuit, that alerts us to feelings of pleasure and happiness, only becomes active during the search for food. The greatest portion of happiness is found in the search and expectations of said emotion.

Major North American studies have revealed that one of the greatest producers of happiness appears when a person feels purpose in their life. Without a clearly defined purpose, seven of every ten individuals feel unsatisfied with their lives. With a purpose, almost the same percent feel satisfied (Lépera).

It is true that as we travel down the path of our live, when we turn and look back, we see that life is full of moments of happiness. There are also murky puddles and muddy trails, but there are the small rays of light from the past and we can decide to hold on to the best moments and leave the less good moments as a positive experience for our growth.

Happy people do not experience constant success, nor do unhappy people experience constant failure. On the contrary, there are studies that demonstrate that both happy and unhappy people tend to have similar experiences in their lives. The difference is that an unhappy person spends on average twice as much time thinking about unpleasant events, while happy people tend to search for thoughts that highlight their personal vision of themselves and to trust in said thoughts (Lyubomirsky).

We are the very actors of the show that is our life, with all those little lights behind us and all those little lights in front of us, that are waiting for us to share moments of happiness. When we are good and we feel happy, there is something within us that radiates outward and towards others…we share our own happiness with them.

"Those that act with courage and bravery will overcome sickness, while those that act with fear will become ill".

(The Yellow Emperor's Internal medicine classic, 500-300 AC)

3.3. KNOWLEDGE

It is important to know where we are from and where we are going. Frequently, people feel lost in this vast and complex world. Knowing our ethnic heritage gives us a great sense of well being, happiness, personal history and a sense of belonging.

> *"Only he who knows himself is capable of directing his own life"*
>
> **(Julius Mwabuki)**

The search for knowledge is never-ending, there is always something new to learn about ourselves, about our past, our present and our future. We need to develop ourselves in all senses to be able to gain access to knowledge.

The pyramid below will help us to gain knowledge of our BEING.

3.3.1. THE PYRAMID

The search for knowledge travels through this pyramid. It allows us to reach the non-duality, the SACRED.

The horizontal path is the path where we develop ourselves both physically and material-wise. We are born, we grow, we study, we work, we buy a house, a car, we have children, a dog…what almost everyone in the world hopes for.

At the same time, the more we develop our SELF, the less we develop our BEING. There are, in reality, two frontiers that impede us from reaching our emotional plan and to develop ourselves. When we are on the horizontal path, we have a vision of TRUTH. The higher we go, we have a broader and broader vision of REALITY.

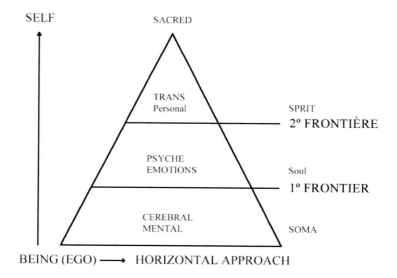

First frontier

    Arrogance

    Pride

False modesty

Second frontier

Acrimony

Resentment

Hate

Vengeance

Non-acceptance

Non-forgiveness

Non-placation

Note: pay attention to traps of attachment, to the environment, to your car, to airplanes…these are MENTAL REFUGES.

HABITS ARE THE IMPULSE OF DEATH!!

SURVIVAL CONTRACT

The survival contract is an oath made unconsciously with yourself, after excessive suffering (sense of failure), during or in the womb. It is a sacred contract made with your BEING and your SELF. The more we construct our personality, the more we fulfill our contract.

However, we must keep in mind that we are faced with a challenge: the psycho-depressive state (we are no longer activated by the energy that comes from the contract). Development on the horizontal level has been completed; we have to balance on the pyramid to develop vertically (spirituality), after having crossed the two frontiers.

3.3.2. THE WORLD OF EMOTIONS

An experience lived is translated on the vegetative nervous system level into physical and emotional manifestations, which are classified as positive or negative. Emotional expressions, both facial and body, are numerous. It's a species of non-verbal communication. Every event has an emotional discharge.

According to traditional Chinese medicine, any excess of emotions (rage-happiness-concern-sadness-fear) can disrupt the energy of the organ related with the emotions experienced. If the energy of an organ is disrupted, the organ will begin to malfunction, with the appearance of symptoms and/or illness.

Connections:

- RAGE – LIVER
- HAPPINESS – HEART
- CONCERN – PANCREAS/SPLEEN
- SADNESS – LUNGS
- FEAR – KIDNEYS

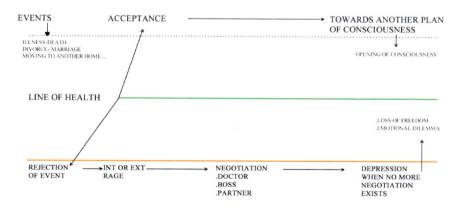

When we take the route downwards (rejection), we form an

emotional dilemma (EMOTIONAL BOILING POT) that flees to the subconscious.

There are as many boiling pots as there are emotional dilemmas.

3.3.3. THE EMOTIONAL BOILING POT AND PSYCHOSOMATIC ESCAPE VALVES

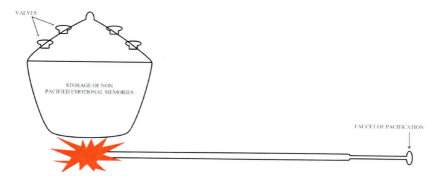

There are many different valves and the role of a therapist is to treat them, balance them and, sometimes, if necessary, eliminate them.

Valve no. 1

- Antibiotics.
- Pain killers
- Anti-inflammatory drugs

BY TAKING THESE SUBSTANCES WE PAINT THE RED LIGHT (symptoms) GREEN (we hide the cause of the problem with medication).

If we block valve no. 1, we will find:

Valve no. 2

Instinctual/drive valve: for example, a person that cannot unwind at work after a stressful day takes it out on their spouse or children, always choosing the weakest member.

Valve no. 3

Sublimation valve (the most sophisticated). Interior energy is transformed in the following:

- Sports, music, painting.
- Refuge in work.
- Reading.
- Spiritual management.
- Smoking.
- Laughing, dancing.

Valve no. 4

Therapeutic valve, used daily in religious traditions.

We become dependent on all things. People can use these safety valves throughout their entire lives. The important thing is to be able to put out the fires as they arise!

PACIFICATION FAUCET: This allows us to reach the other side of the mirror and see reality. After valve no. 4, life takes over to calm different emotional dilemmas by means of different systems or mediums.

3.3.4. BEHAVIOR

"The mind is the origin of everything"

(Buddhist Sutra)

There are four possible attitudes that we can have for all events in our lives.

1st The non-recognition of the emotional dilemma   **SELF**
Discomfort/uneasiness.
Distress.
Phobias.

2nd Late/delayed recognition
Discomfort/uneasiness ++
Fleeing from the present due to anticipation.
Depression.

3rd Instant recognition
Discomfort/uneasiness +++
Devalued subconscious self-image.

4th Free behavior   **BEING**
To let one's guard down.
Smile. ⟶ pacification phase

3.3.5. THE FREEDOM SPIRAL

Going through the phases of this spiral, one by one, is necessary to become free from an emotional dilemma.

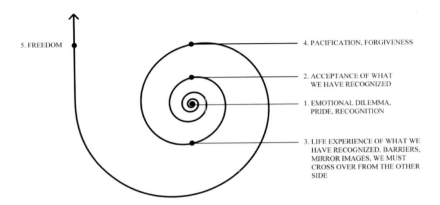

3.4. COINCIDENCES

"When man lost contact with magic…he called it coincidence"

(J.L. Parise)

It is more than obvious that coincidences do not exist. Things do not happen just because, everything happens for a reason. Of course, it is not easy to accept destiny in some circumstances…

But I do not want to talk about misfortune…

An example:

You are reading my book right now. A few days ago you would not have thought about reading this book but yet you are now reading it. Within a few days, after finishing this book, you will ask yourself the following questions: was it foreseen that I would read this book?

You do not have many alternative responses: of course! Because you read it!

Scheduled? Misfortune? Coincidence? At random?

Therefore, life is only made of coincidences (that, in reality, are not coincidences at all).

"Tao originates all things"

(Lao Tse, "Tao Te King")

I am convinced that there is an energy that makes things "the way they are". We need our learning experiences to evolve to another level of conscience.

3.5. EXCUSES

"The essential nature of every human being is perfect and impeccable, but after years of immersion in the world, we easily forget our roots and adopt a false nature"

(Lao-tsé)

A common saying is that old habits die hard, which implies that changing thought patterns that have been established long ago is nearly impossible. This system consists of a long list of explanations and defenses that can be summarized into one single word: excuses.

Said habits come from our education, from our parents, from life events. These have installed themselves inside of us without allowing us any space for critical thought or the power to decide if we want them or not. At the same time, you truly can change your habits.

To be able to change them, first you have to recognize them. They are like a virus that enter in your computer and make it function in a manner that is uncomfortable to you. And just as you clean a computer, we can also uninstall a habit that dominates you.

One of the excuses is genetic, "my genes are the culprit". However, it has been scientifically demonstrated that during gestation in our mother's abdomens, with the passing of time and life experiences, our original DNA, which is inherited from our parents, partially changes. Approximately 95% of people have no genetic cause of illness, depression or any other disorder.

The other typical excuse is rooted in early childhood and family conditioning that influences you in so many ways.

"It is surely impossible to say that change always means improvement, but I can say is that all improvement needs change"

(G.C. Lichtenberg)

According to Wayne W. Dyer, the 18 most frequent excuses and affirmations that will help you to eliminate them are listed below:

1. It will be difficult. I am able to perform any task that I put my mind to, with ease and comfort.

2. It will be risky. Being myself implies no risk. It is my original truth and I live it without fear.

3. It is going to take a long time. I have infinite patience when dealing with fulfilling my destiny.

4. There will be family drama. I prefer them to hate me for who I am than for them to love me for who I am not.

5. I do not deserve it. I am a divine creation, a fragment of the universe, and therefore, I deserve it.

6. It is not my nature. My essential nature is perfect and impeccable. I always must return to this nature.

7. I cannot allow it for myself. I am connected to a source of unlimited abundance.

8. Nobody is going to help me. The adequate circumstances and adequate people are already there and they will appear to me over time.

9. It has never happened before. I am willing to attract all that I desire, starting here and now.

10. I am not strong enough. I have access to unlimited help. My strength comes from my connection with the source of my Being.

11. I am not smart enough. I am a creation of a divine mind, everything is perfect, and I am a genius of my own right.

12. I am too old (or too young). I am an infinite being. The age of my body does not influence what I do today or who I am.

13. Rules do not allow me to do it. I live my life following divine rules.

14. It is too big. I only think about what I can do now. Thinking small, I achieve big things.

15. I do not have enough energy. I am passionate about my life, and this passion fills me with enthusiasm and energy.

16. I feel guilt from my personal family history. I live in the present moment and I am thankful for all of my vital experiences from my childhood.

17. I am too busy. When I organize my life, I am free to respond to the calling of my soul.

18. I am afraid. I can achieve anything that I put my mind to, because I know I am never alone.

"Do not let yourself be reigned by sadness, do not abandon yourself to dark thoughts. The happiness of the heart is the life of man, contentment is what makes the days longer"

(Ecclesiastes, 30)

3.6. CREATING YOUR REALITY

Almost all of us know about the power of intention. Thought goes further than one can imagine. The law of attraction is a universal law for all.

All of our thoughts, positive or negative, influence our daily lives. Thought also influence material.

Dr. Masaru Emoto, a Japanese researcher, has shared his astonishing research on the consciousness of water in "messages from water". His experiments consisted of writing pleasant words on paper and pasting them in containers of water. "Love and appreciation", "thank you", caused positive changes in the crystals of the water where they were placed, orienting itself in a harmonious and homogeneous manner, while "I hate you and I will kill you" made the molecules of the same frozen water "emit" unharmonious messages.

It is found, once more, at the base of this research, that more than 70% of our body and the planet earth consist of the same material: $H2O$. We can sense that the physical disorder of negative thoughts toward another person or being could cause...

A world without thoughts is unthinkable. Everything starts with a desire. Creating means desiring. Even the desire to not desire is a desire. Every process of creation starts with a desire, an idea.

This idea is energy. Verbal information must be added to this energy.

"...in the beginning was the Word..." (Logos)

(First chapter of the Gospel of John)

"Tao", the Primordial Essence that is present before any thing exists, means just that "To speak". Everything starts with the word, everything is set in motion by speech.

"Logos" also means "Light", and light exists to be projected. Projecting oneself in the future is visualizing the result of what we desire.

All civilizations of the world, far away and at different times, followed the same rituals, the same steps to create their own reality.

José Luis Parise clearly explains this in his book "CASUALIZAR" (to create coincidences). I recommend reading this book to anyone that is prepared to create their own reality.

This is why it is so important to have positive thoughts to created coincidences!!

3.7. RECOMMENDATIONS

"The interior strength of each one of us is the most important and strongest curing agent"

(Hippocrates)

3.7.1. REJUVENATE YOUR BRAIN

Many companies invest in intellectual training. There are many alternatives to exercise our neurons that are available to us.

- Mental training: crossword puzzles, sudokus, word search puzzles...
- New learning experiences: learn a new language, music, reading...
- Find new hobbies: travel, opera, taking walks...
- Exercise regularly: remember "a healthy mind in a healthy body".
- Do leisure activities with your family or friends.
- Develop your creativity: draw, dance, sing...
- Learn to relax and be quiet: tai chi, chi kung, yoga...

"Silence is a source of great strength"

(Lao Tse)

3.7.2. AFFIRMATIONS

The following are types of affirmations that I recommend to repeat to ourselves and constantly verbalize for them to be a part of our reality:

> I am tranquil. I am at peace inside and out.
> I am healthy, I feel good.
> I am one with the infinite power of the universe.
> I have the strength to change my life in a positive manner.
> Happiness is my birthright. I am happy.
> A place under the sun belongs to me. I claim it.
> Universe, you are perfect, I am made in your image, I am perfect.
> I am perfectly fine without smoking.
> I feel good when I exercise.

3.7.3. AVOID

Situations that cause us distress or uneasiness should be limited as much as possible.

Avoid:

Situations that drain our energy or harm others and us.

Fights.

Yelling.

Getting angry.

Insults and all kind of negative expressions.

Judging others.

Prejudices.

Spending time with negative people…

3.7.4. PERSONAL LIFE PHILOSOPHY

"Is there a more valued good than health for mankind?"

(Socrates)

A personal life philosophy means to possess a group of personal thoughts, beliefs and values that help us to direct our lives along the path of health, peace and happiness.

These thoughts are at the base of our motivation and the fuel for our actions.

A smart life philosophy will show us how to use our energy and time to achieve things that are truly important to us.

I have listed a few concepts that can help to enrich your life philosophy below:

"Nothing lasts forever, this too shall pass." (popular saying).
I can overcome any problem.
Everything is relative.
"Every cloud has a silver lining" (popular saying).
"Everything is vanity" (Ecclesiastes).
"Letting go, everything is done by itself" (popular Spanish saying).
When money is lost, nothing is lost.
When health is lost, something is lost.
When peace is lost, everything is lost.
"I spend more than half of my life worrying about things that never happened" (Winston Churchill).
Not one of my patients was cured without directing their spirituality" (Carl Jung".
"Adapt like water" (Asian saying).
"If you value your life, you value your time, as that is what it is made of" (Benjamin Franklin).
"Do what's right, come what may" (popular saying).

A smile costs nothing but gives so much.
"Things are as important as we make them" (popular saying).

3.7.5. PERSONAL PEACE

The following suggestions were created by an anonymous psychologist that wrote them for his/her own personal peace.

Organize your mind to be at peace. Accentuate all that is positive and concentrate on the good.

Do everything the best that you can, anywhere and anytime.

Do not take yourself too seriously.

Do not compare yourself or compete with anyone else; do not allow for anyone else to establish your rules.

Be the best that is possible. If your neighbor needs help, give it to him; if not, leave him to his own free will.

Do not be envious or hold on to resentment, this wasted energy and harms your health.

Leave your home and get together with others, greet others, take the initiative to say "hello", make others happy and you will also be happy.

Do not hold on to old grudges or resentment. Use your memory only to remember good things.

Keep busy, performing constructive tasks. Help others that need help, this will bring great benefits to your well being.

Speak to the universe with an attitude of gratitude, thanking it for all that you have. We all want peace, profound peace. We must start within ourselves.

3.7.6. AMARANTA METHOD

The Amaranta Method is the fruit of a deep investigation and experimentation that was led with the intention of healing completely and permanently that which we have been dragging along with us for thousands of years of darkness on all levels. Through channelings, a path for spiritual growth was designed (the Amaranta Path), as well as an energetic healing method, so that those who feel it in their heart may get in touch with their Inner Master and manifest its presence in their life.

This tool of light can be used to perform therapies and courses. The therapies are meant to heal traumas, conflicts, illnesses, past lives, problems related to the family tree, to the inner child, the maternal womb, mental patterns, bonds, decrees from the collective unconscious, etc. There are different types of courses in which we learn how to work with The Method to perform healings, cleanses and powerful activations among others. For more information, visit www.metodoamaranta.com

CHAPTER II

FOOD INTOLERANCES

1. FOOD INTOLERANCES

1.1. WHAT ARE INTOLERANCES? HOW DO THEY AFFECT US?

1.1.1. INTOLERANCE AND ALLERGIES, DIFFERENT CONCEPTS

A food intolerance is the abnormal response of our body to a certain type of food, coloring or preservative (additive) without activating our immune system. It is therefore a phenomenon that has nothing to do with allergies or food sensitivities.

The principal difference is that intolerance to a food triggers a metabolic response; allergies, on the other hand, imply an immune system reaction against a substance that the organism recognizes as harmful.

POSSIBLE ANOMALOUS INTERACTIONS BETWEEN THE ORGANISM AND FOODS.

Toxic:

Foods in poor condition: salmonella, etc.

Non-toxic:

Responses where the immune system intervenes with antibodies (Ig):

- Food allergies: IgE
- Food sensitivity: IgG

Responses without the intervention of the immune system that are only detected through a CYTOTOXICITY test: FOOD INTOLERANCE.

There is an anomalous reaction in food intolerances where pro-inflammatory immunochemicals are secreted such as prostaglandins, interleukins, leukotrienes, etc., that act remotely on the "target" cells, causing

symptoms to appear.

DIFFERENCES BETWEEN ALLERGIES AND INTOLERANCES

Frequency of appearance.

Food intolerances are ten times more frequent than allergies.

Latent period and sensitization.

An allergy needs a first contact to become sensitized to the allergen. There is no latent period in food intolerances.

Appearance of symptoms.

Allergies are immediate.

Food intolerances take place up to 72 hours later.

Intensity of symptoms.

Allergies: allergy symptoms can be severe, leading to anaphylactic shock and even death.

Food intolerances: mild to chronic symptoms.

Incidence of foods and additives.

Allergies: fundamentally milk, egg and nuts.

Food intolerances: to almost any product:

- Additives 17%
- Fruit 16%
- Nuts 14%
- Dairy-eggs 13%
- Vegetables 9%
- Fish 8%
- Meat 7%
- Legumes 5%
- Shellfish 4%
- Other 7%

At-risk foods.

From research on food intolerances, the following foods have been recognized as at-risk: WHEAT, EGGS, MILK, YEASTY, SUGAR,

CHOCOLATE, COFFEE, CABBAGE, TOMATO, POTATO, STRAWBERRIES, BANANAS, BARLEY, CORN AND BEEF.

1.1.2. ADDITIVES: PRESERVATIVES AND ARTIFICIAL COLORING

WHAT IS A FOOD ADDITIVE?

Legally, an additive is considered as any substance added to foods to improve their physical properties, flavor, that helps to extend its shelf life or presentation, which enhances the food's natural color and keeps its qualities for longer.

Although associated with modern times, food additives have been used for centuries. They have been used since man learned to preserve foods from the harvest for the following year and to preserve meat and fish with salting and smoking techniques.

The Egyptians used artificial coloring and aromas to enhance certain foods, and the Romans used brine (potassium nitrate), spices and artificial coloring to preserve and improve the appearance of foods.

Cooks have frequently used powdered yeast that makes certain foods grow, thickeners for sauces and artificial coloring, such as the cochineal, to transform high quality raw material into safe, healthy and appetizing foods.

In general, the purpose of traditional home cooking and of the food industry, which use methods of elaboration to prepare and preserve foods, is the same.

According to norms defined by the countries of the European Union, all authorized food additives correspond to a code, formed by the letter E followed by a three or four digit number. Each code identifies the chemical name, the color, the group, the use in foods and its properties.

Spain, as with the rest of the European Union, has very strict legislation regarding the additives that can be used (excluding various), the foods to which they can be added, the maximum content allowed and the purity required of said additives.

There are additives allowed in Spain and not in others, such as E123 prohibited in the United States, or E239 prohibited in France. More research must be done and the criteria of possible side effects that are harmful to health should be unified regarding all food additives. The corresponding official organisms, when authorizing the use of a specific additive, take into account that said additive is an addition to the correct processing of the foods and not an agent to mask deficient sanitary or technological handling conditions or a system to defraud the consumer, tricking them about the true freshness of a food.

The list of the most used additives in foods that can cause some kind of intolerance is found below. Legally, if multinational food companies use them, it must be specified on the product packaging:

ADDITIVE	**ARTIFICIAL COLORING**
(E200) SORBIC ACID	(E102) TARTRAZINE
(E210) BENZOIC ACID	(E104) QUINOLINE YELLOW
(E221) SODIUM SULPHITE	(E110) SUNSET YELLOW FCF
(E223) SODIUM METABISULPHITE	(E123) AMARANTH
(E249) POTASSIUM NITRITE	(E124) BRILLIANT SCARLET
(E252) POTASSIUM NITRATE	(E127) ERYTHROSINE
(E433) POLYSORBATE 80	(E131) PATENT BLUE
(E621) MONOSODIUM GLUTAMATE	(E132) INDIGO CARMINE
(E951) ASPARTAME	(E142) GREEN
(E954) SACCHARIN	(E151) BRILLIANT BLACK

1.2. DO I HAVE ANY FOOD INTOLERANCES?

When we eat a food to which we are intolerant, a certain level of toxicity is generated in our cells that cause numerous symptoms.

Feeling a great urge to eat a certain food, and never feeling satiated even after eating it is a type of intolerance that can be defined as a "food dependence".

Ninety percent of the adult population suffers from some kind of food intolerance, and the number of intolerances increases with age.

Food intolerances are ten times as frequent as food allergies. In the ranking of food intolerances, additives are first followed by fruits and vegetables.

Many people are not aware that they suffer from food intolerance as the reaction is not always immediate. Symptoms may appear two or three days after eating that specific food in many cases.

Fruits and vegetables tend to be the star foods for weight-loss diets, foods that appear high up in the food intolerance ranking. This is the reason that in spite of correctly following the diet, many times we do not lose the weight that we would like to.

Make your food your best medicine. By correcting our food intolerances we can reduce chronic symptoms, and recover feelings of good health, energy and vitality.

1.3. PHYSIOPATHOLOGY OF INTOLERANCES

1.3.1. INTESTINAL DYSBIOSIS

Intestinal dysbiosis is a dysfunction where the permeability of the intestinal membrane and flora are altered.

Over-eating, the lack of eating different foods, and, sometimes, genetics, are responsible for these alterations.

1.3.2. FUNCTIONS OF INTESTINAL FLORA

Metabolic:

Fermentation.

Putrefaction.

Synthesis of certain vitamins and enzymes.

Favors absorption of calcium, magnesium and iron.

Stabilization of intestinal pH.

Nutritional:

Growth and differentiation of epithelial cells.

Protective:

Synthesis of bacteriocins (many times considered as narrow spectrum antibiotics).

1.3.3. COMPOSITION OF INTESTINAL FLORA

We can classify the most typical genus and species of the bacteria based on their primary function in our intestines.

Protective:

Lactobacillus.
Bifidobacterium.
Bacteroides.

Immunomodulatory:

Enterococcus.
E. coli.

Proteolytic

Escherichia coli Biovare.
Proteus.
Klebsiella.
Pseudomona.
Clostridium.
Enterobacter.
Citrobacter.

Fungus and yeasts.

1.3.4. CAUSES OF DYSBIOSIS

Environmental factors.

Stress.
Environmental contamination.
Pesticides.

Diet.

Insufficient chewing of foods.
Malnutrition and shortage/lack of vitamins and minerals.
Pro-inflammatory diet.

Intrinsic factors.

Deficit of hydrochloric acid and pancreatic enzymes.

Alterations of intestinal motility.
Aging.

Extrinsic factors.

Systemic diseases: cerebral trauma, epilepsy, burns, stress, rheumatoid arthritis, celiac disease, neoplasms.

Medication and other treatments.
Non-steroid anti-inflammatory drugs.
Corticosteroids.
Antibiotics.
Chemo- and radiotherapy.

Intestinal infections.

From bacteria (salmonellosis…).
From parasites (tapeworms…).
From fungus.
From viruses: rotavirus, reovirus, adenovirus, HIV.

1.3.5. CONSEQUENCES OF DYSBIOSIS

Increase of intestinal permeability.

Immune system alterations.

Chronic fatigue and fibromyalgia.

Inflammation/intestinal neoplasms.

Obesity.

Depression.

Hyperactivity.

1.3.6. CONSEQUENCES OF THE ALTERATION OF INTESTINAL PERMEABILITY

When the barrier of permeability is altered, in poor condition or insufficient, the interstitial space is left vulnerable to the entrance of:

Pathogenic germs;
Allergens;
Harmful substances;
Undigested foods.

As a result, there is a predisposition to certain disease and severe intestinal discomfort.

1.4. SYMPTOMS ASSOCIATED WITH FOOD INTOLERANCES

Symptoms may be greatly varied and affect any apparatus or system of our body. In most cases, medical staff fails to relate the symptoms to a food intolerance, however, it has been found that when certain foods are removed from the patient's daily diet, the symptoms completely or mostly disappear.

General symptoms:

Fatigue, water retention, bags under eyes, post-prandial tiredness, bad breath, increased sweating, hair loss.

Nervous system:

Headaches, anxiety, depression, irritability, memory problems, difficulties concentrating, vertigo, hot flashes.

Respiratory apparatus:

Difficulties breathing, stuffy nose, asthma, cough, allergic rhinitis, sinusitis.

Cardio-circulatory apparatus:

Blood pressure alterations, palpitations, premature ventricular contractions, increase of blood coagulation properties.

Digestive apparatus:

Bloating, nausea, abdominal pain and cramping, gastritis, colitis, bowel disorders (diarrhea, constipation), gasses, anal pruritus, hemorrhoids.

Uro-genital apparatus:

Cystitis, uro-genital swelling, premenstrual syndrome.

Musculoskeletal system:

Cramping, spasms, trembling of muscles, muscular weakness, joint pain, carpal tunnel syndrome, arthritis, swelling of muscles and tendons.

Epidermis:

Localized and generalized pruritus, acne, eczema, dermatitis, various types of dermatological lesions, psoriasis.

Aesthetic alterations:

Cellulitis, overweight, obesity.

1.5. TREATMENT

The determination of intolerances is done with a blood test (FOOD INTOLERANCE TEST), where blood cells are placed in contact with different foods and additives and their response is evaluated (CYTOTOXICITY).

Intolerant foods will be catalogued according to the level of toxicity. According to Dr. Marchetti Rita, of the Nutrition Center of Rome, there are four levels of reactions. However, a low level reaction, for example, level 1, can cause the same severe symptoms in the organism as a higher reaction. Therefore, regardless of the level of the reaction, avoiding said food will be necessary.

A negative reaction is when the structure of the red and white blood cells along with the platelets remains unaltered.

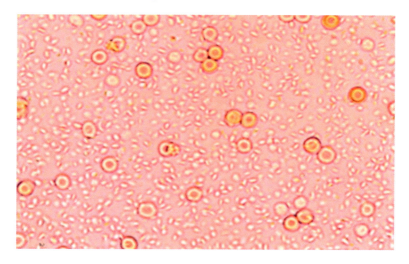

Level 1: the element reacts with a platelet aggression and must be eliminated from the diet for one to two months.

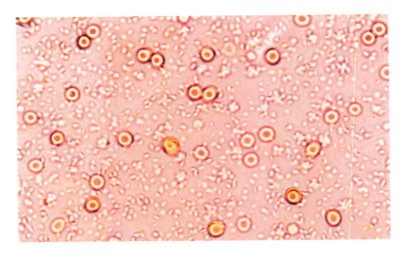

Level 2: the element has harmed approximately 25% of the white blood cells and must be eliminated from the diet for two to three months.

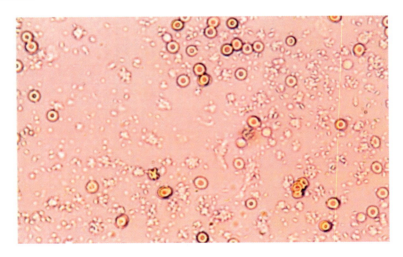

Level 3: the element has harmed approximately 50% of the white blood cells and must be eliminated from the diet for three to four months.

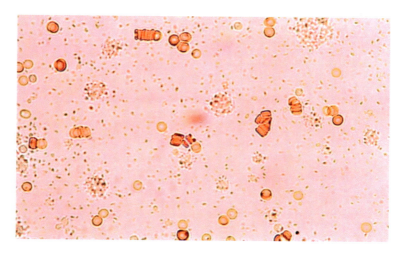

Level 4: the element has harmed approximately 50% of the white blood cells, as well as partial damage to the red blood cells, and must be eliminated from the diet for six months.

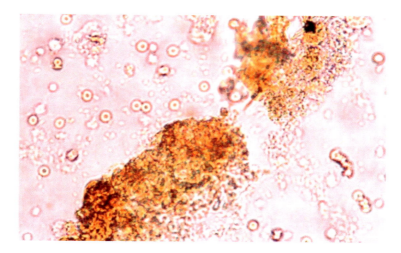

This way, we can truly know which foods are those that do not sit well with us, and thus be able to create a completely personalized diet. The elimination of retained liquids and the increase of vital energy are the first effects that we notice when the foods that we are intolerant to are removed from our diet.

ATTENTION

Many laboratories offer some kind of food intolerance testing. When they are asked which parameters they evaluate or measure, their response is the antibodies IgG or IgE. That is, that it is not truly food intolerance testing but food sensitivity or allergy testing, where the immune system intervenes. This is not the same thing!!

The first step in treatment is to have a clinical history taken and a thorough diagnosis made for each patient, taking into account their lifestyle and habits. Once we have the results of the test, and after a therapist's interpretation, treatment should be directed from various angles:

1.5.1. ELIMINATION OF CAUSES:

Intolerant foods: intolerant foods are removed for at least three months. Possible nutritional shortages of certain basic nutrients must be evaluated and alternatives must be found. The diet should be reorganized according to correct associations;

Irritating foods: such as alcohol, tea, coffee, fried foods and an excess of red meat, anti-inflammatory drugs, etc. Moderate to no consumption of these products is recommended during this same period;

Chewing and swallowing guidelines:

"Chew solid food until it is liquid and swallow liquids as if they were solids"

(Chinese proverb)

A person that does not chew their food enough swallows air, causing gasses and bloating. Chewing is the first step of digestion, to decompose foods. Poorly chewed foods reach the stomach without having been crushed, with the following consequences:

- The digestive process is lengthened;
- Difficulty absorbing nutrients from foods;
- Imbalance of intestinal flora and alterations of the mucus membranes are favored.
- Indigestion
- Excessive production of gasses.
- Also, poor chewing can provoke:
- Eating more than necessary, stomach bloating.
- Not enjoying meals as flavors and textures are hardly noticed.

1.5.2. CLEANSING OF TOXINS: DETOXIFICATION AND DRAINAGE.

This treatment consists of cleansing the extracellular matrix of toxins generated by:

- The consumption of intolerant foods;
- Residues generated from a poor diet;
- Taking medication;
- Environmental toxicity;
- Pesticides;
- Viral or bacterial infections;
- Toxic metabolites from our own metabolism.

Detoxification therapy will be carried out with homeopathy and under the close supervision of a health professional, using the following:

- SCROPHULARIA CPTO (DROPS).
- BERBERIS-SOLIDAGO (DROPS).
- NUX VOMICA M.P. (DROPS).

DILUTE 10 DROPS OF EACH IN ONE AND A HALF LITERS OF WATER AND DRINK THROUGHOUT THE DAY, FOR ONE WEEK. IF YOU DO NOT EXPERIENCE ANY DISCOMFORT, ADD ONE MORE DROP OF EACH EVERY DAY UNTIL YOU REACH 30 DROPS OF EACH, AND MAINTAIN AT THIS LEVEL FOR 8 TO 10 WEEKS.

1.5.3. EQUILIBRIUM OF INTESTINAL FLORA

We need to repopulate the intestinal flora that was destroyed by all the previously mentioned phenomena. Adding prebiotics and probiotics to our diet will provide beneficial effects in different areas:

- Stimulation of the immune system.
- Prevention of diarrhea and constipation.

- Improved digestion of lactose.
- Collaboration of pre- and probiotics in the synthesis of vitamins and fatty acids.
- Lowered pH in the intestines.
- Inhibited growth of pathogenic bacteria.
- Improved the availability of minerals and promotes the correct absorption of calcium, magnesium and iron.

I recommend taking LIFE 9 from Young Living

1.5.4. REPAIR AND PROTECTION OF THE INTESTINAL MEMBRANE: L-GLUTAMINE

The long-term dysbiosis leaves the intestinal membrane unprotected, with the previously-mentioned consequences. For this reason, once the intestinal flora is repopulated, we have to protect and seal the intestinal membrane through the ingestion of L-GLUTAMINE, an amino acid. This can be easily taken in capsule form or drink daily 30 ml of NINGXIA RED by Young Living.

1.5.5. REINTRODUCTION OF FOODS

After evaluating renal clearance, and taking into account the progress of the patient's symptoms, we can start to reintroduce the foods to which they were intolerant, starting with the least toxic and following with those of intermediate toxicity. Consuming those that were found to be highly toxic is not recommended.

Guidelines to be followed:

- Eat the food or an additive one day.
- Wait 72 hours (3 days) and observe to see if any symptoms appear. If they do, wait another month to reintroduce said food or additive.
- If no symptoms appear, eat said food or additive again and

wait another 72 hours.

Evaluation:

If not symptoms appear:

- Cleared;

- Move on to the next food.

If any symptoms appear:

- Remove from diet again;

- Try again in one month.

1.5.6. INTAKE OF NUTRIENTS FOR OPTIMAL ABSORPTION AND METABOLISM

Currently, ortho-molecular medicine is very helpful for the metabolism. Epidemiologically speaking, it has been demonstrated that the intake of antioxidant vitamins reduces the risk of suffering from the following ailments:

- Cancer;

- Cardiovascular diseases;

- Cataracts.

Depending on the therapist's evaluation, the following will be prescribed:

- Vitamins (respecting their synergies);

- Essential fatty acids;

- Glucosamine, chondroitin sulfate;

- Digestive enzymes;

- Amino acids;

- Algae…

I CAN ENSURE YOU THAT WHEN OUR HABITS AND OUR FOOD INTOLERANCES ARE CORRECTED, MANY OF THE CHRONIC SYMPTOMS THAT WE SUFFER WILL BE REDUCED AND WE WILL FEEL NOTICEABLE MORE ENERGETIC AND VITAL, AND OVERALL HEALTHIER.

THE EXPERIENCE OF THOUSANDS OF PATIENTS, AS WELL AS MY OWN EXPERIENCE AND THAT OF MANY OF MY FAMILY MEMBERS AND CLOSE FRIENDS CONFIRM MY METHOD.

CHAPTER III

ALTERNATIVE MEDICINE

1. INTRODUCTION

My philosophy is that patients must be treated holistically; by rebalancing the mechanical, energetic, functional and emotional aspects of each person. The different therapies that follow serve as a guide to patients, so that they can find balance in all different aspects of their lives.

1.1. MECHANICAL REBALANCING

1.1.1. OSTEOPATHY

Osteopathy is a soft medicine that consists of treating disorders by manipulating vertebrae, joints, the cranium and internal organs.

Osteopathy is based on the notion that all systems of the body work together (all are related to each other) and, therefore, the malfunctioning or disorders that affect one system may affect the functioning or others.

Osteopathic treatment, which is called manipulation, consists of a system of practical techniques geared towards alleviating pain, restoring function and promoting health and well being.

It uses a wide array of techniques (high velocity and short amplitude pulses, functional, visceral, cranial, gynecological techniques, etc.) to return the body to its natural harmony and equilibrium that avoid diseases and impede recovery.

By means of manipulation of the muscular-skeletal, visceral and cranial systems, conditions or diseases of vital organs can be cured as this manipulation will help to revitalize blood flow or return joints to their normal degree of mobility and, therefore, cure the patient.

Osteopathy claims that the body suffers from subluxations, that is, small displacements in the spinal vertebrae that compress nerves. The effect of this is that the body's tissues and organs deteriorate and a poor connection is generated between the brain and the spine causing pain and disease.

1.1.2. TYPES OF OSTEOPATHY

Joint osteopathy: This type is dedicated to the restoration of the muscular-skeletal apparatus and posture, focusing on the spine and joints.

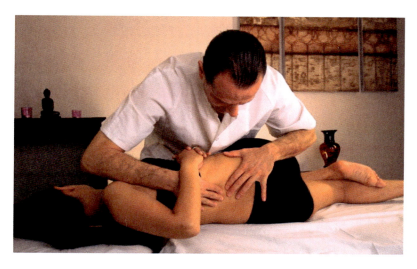

Cranial osteopathy: focused on cranial problems and their influence on the central nervous system.

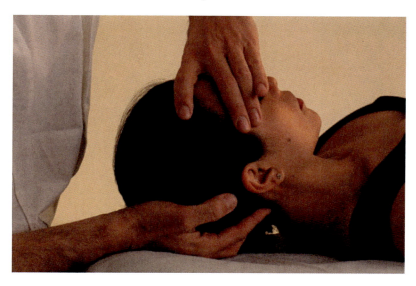

Visceral osteopathy: focused on curing organs and the genital apparatus, improving their function through manipulation to achieve better blood flow.

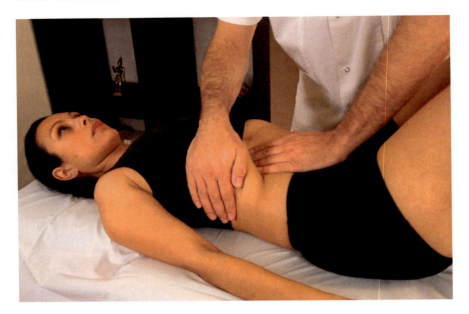

1.2. ENERGETIC REBALANCING
1.1.2. TRADITIONAL CHINESE MEDICINE

At the beginning, the universe was in a state of "Wu Chi" (that means "emptiness", "there is nothing"). Like a sphere full of a "sea of air", it started to move itself, always changing.

Water was produced from said movement (from the theory of the five elements). Fire warmed the "sea of air" (this "sphere"), and a great explosion took place (Big Bang?).

From this explosion the cleanest and lightest particles rose to the sky: Yang. The dirtiest and heaviest particles descended towards earth: Yin. Between the sky and earth, man and nature existed. This is how the principle of Yin-Yang is defined in the Trigram concept: Earth-Man-Sky.

"When the Chi of the earth rises in the form of clouds; when the Chi of the sky descends, rain is produced". Like day and night, hot and cold, movement and stillness.

"The movement and changes of the Yin/Yang promote things to development and change". This is the explanation found in the chapter "The Manifestations of Yin and Yang" of Suwen, the interdependence between opposing and complementary forces. The universe expands.

The most basic force of the universe that makes material structures dynamic in traditional Chinese medicine is called Chi. Traditional Chinese medicine, also known simple as Chinese medicine or traditional oriental medicine, is the common name given to a wide range of traditional medical practices developed in China throughout its millenary cultural evolution.

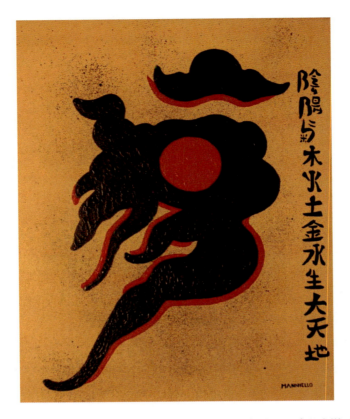

This medicine is based on the concept of balanced "chi" (or vital energy), that courses through our bodies. Chi regulates spiritual, emotional, mental and physical balance. It turns into matter but its essence is invisible. We only see the expression of said essence (that is found in the macrocosm, the universe, as well as in microcosms, our body).

The life of man is the result of the concentration of energy. If energy is concentrated, life appears. If energy is dispersed, death survives.

The Yin-Yang theory, the theory of the five elements, Zang-Fu (organs), essence, Chi, blood (Xue), body fluids, meridians (energy channels), etiology, pathogenesis, diagnostic systems, and prevention and treatment regimens, are the fundamental pillars for good health and a long life.

According to traditional Chinese medicine, disease occurs when the Chi flow is altered and an imbalance of the Yin and Yang takes place.

The components of this type of medicine include herbal therapies and diet, physical exercise that reconstitutes health, meditation, acupuncture and restorative massages.

1.2.2. ACUPUNCTURE

Acupuncture is a medical discipline that is one of the tools used in traditional Chinese medicine. It consists of puncturing certain areas of the body, found at the "meridians", with special needles, to balance energy.

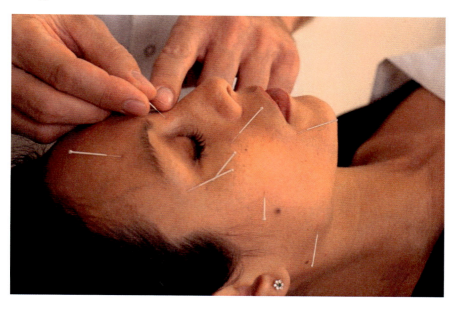

Its origins are estimated to be from 5,000 years ago. The oldest writings (NEI-JING) are dated 2,000 years ago. In 443 A.C., Korean doctors contributed this knowledge to Japan.

At the end of the 17th century, Jesuit missionaries and doctors from the Dutch East India Company introduced their observations from Chinese medicine into the West. Soulié de Morant introduced them to France at the end of the 19th century.

1.2.3. REIKI

The term "reiki" is a Japanese word. REI means "universal" and refers to the scope and nature of this practice, and KI means "energy", and thus the word "reiki" can be understood as the universal vital energy. It is an alternative therapy as it is intended to cure through the approximation of the hands of the practitioner to the body of the receiver in order to transfer "universal energy" to them.

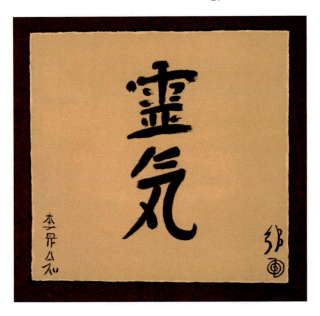

What is reiki?

Reiki is a natural curing method that uses universal vital energy to cure physical and mental diseases.

Mikao Usui, a Japanese monk, developed reiki during a spiritual retreat half-way through the 19th century, although he always reiterated the he merely "rediscovered" a millenary curing technique that already existed but must have been forgotten for many, many years.

The practice of reiki is based on an emitter or channel that, through their hands, transmits reiki (vital energy) to a receiver, that can be him or herself, or another person, in order to palliate or eliminate maladies or diseases. However, given that reiki is universal energy, treatments can also be directed to other living beings such as animals or even plants.

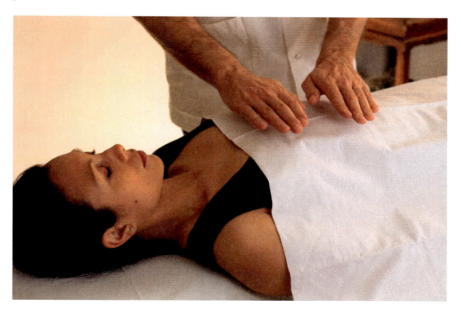

The reiki method is based on Hindu beliefs about chakras, which would explain the states of health of human beings. According to these beliefs, the malfunctioning or blockage of one or various chakras would cause or aggravate the poor state of health leading to diseases and disorders. The method consists of directing reiki energy to the chakras of the ill person (receiver), unblocking them and fortifying the recovery process of the receiver.

The five principles of reiki: Doctor Mikao Usui established

guidelines for life for reiki based on the principles of Emperor Meiji, and invited his students to follow them. A more literal translation of the original document in Japanese where these principles are written is found below:

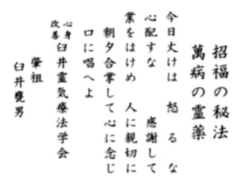

"Just today,

don't get mad,

don't worry,

give thanks,

work honestly,

be kind.

Do Gassho meditation in the morning and at night".

1.3. FUNCTIONAL REBALANCING

1.3.1. AYURVEDIC MEDICINE

Ayurveda is an ancient Hindu health science that comes from Hindu traditions, a wide and extensive written tradition described in the Vedas, the oldest texts known to humanity, where the knowledge not only of medical science but also other sciences such as mathematics, astrology, psychology, language, etc. are found.

Practiced in the East from Tibet to Siberia over the last five thousand years, it is originally from Siberia according to research, and it spread to the East through the Mongols thousands of years ago.

Ayurvedic medicine (which means "science of life") is a comprehensive medicine system that combines natural therapies with a highly personalized approach to the treatment of diseases.

The key to ayurvedic medicine is the "Constitution" (Prakriti), and once identified, said Constitution allows us to establish a total profile of an individual's health. The subtle and intricate constitutional profile of an individual is the first critical step of this process, that once identified, will be the base of all clinical decisions.

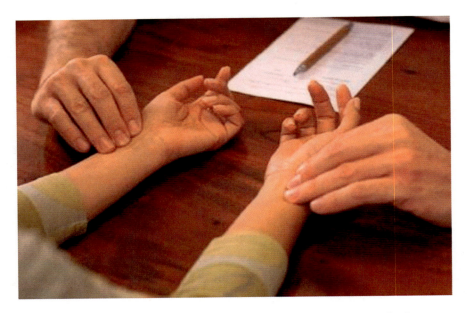

Ayurvedic medicine is based on the concept of the metabolic types of the body, or the dosha. The three metabolic types of the body are known as vata, pitta and kapha. It has its own precise diagnostic system.

Ayurvedic medicine holds that for health to be reestablished, the physical or emotional disease or imbalance must first be correctly diagnosed. Afterwards, there are four primary methods that a ayurvedic doctor uses to manage the disease: cleansing and detoxification, palliation, rejuvenation (rasayana) and mental hygiene.

1.3.2. CONNECTIVE TISSUE REFLEX THERAPY: THE E. DICKE METHOD

In 1889 the English doctors HEAD and MACKENZIE established a relationship between sick organs and the skin. They claimed that from one single disease, the same cutaneous territory presents hypersensitivity.

In 1929, Ms. Elisabeth DICKE (physical therapist), confirmed that manifestations of a pathological phenomena existed at the subcutaneous tissue level. The following tissue-level modifications were observed: sclerosis, swelling and retractions. She thus elaborated a special technique that consists of stretching and displacing the skin from its original place, starting with the non-sensitive regions. Surprising results were obtained using this technique with various pathologies.

Since 1960, scientific research to theoretically justify the reflex technique and its practical applications was carried out by the INSTITUT E. DICKE DE BINDEGEWEBSTHÉRAPIE (reflex massage of connective tissues) in BRUSSELS (Dr. KLEIN, Melle HENDRICKX (physical therapist), to whom we owe the development of this technique that has been scientifically validated).

1.3.2.1. NEURAL THERAPY PRINCIPLES

All sick organs can project themselves to the periphery of the body through the corresponding reflexive nerve pathways in the metameres (territories).

A metamere is a territory of innervation of one single spinal nerve, from where it comes out of the neural foramen to the small parcel of tissue that innervates it.

The neural therapy acts on the periphery of the body to reach the organ through nerve pathways.

1.3.2.2. MEANS OF ACTION

With the middle and ring fingertips, pressure is applied to the skin while stretching it, generating a nerve impulse.

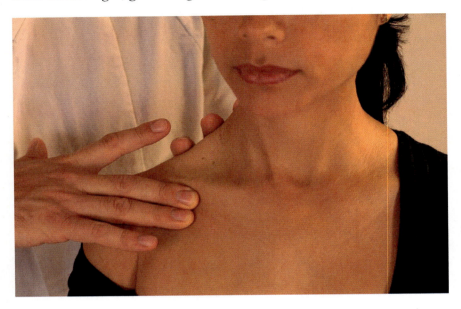

Through vegetative innervation, action takes place on all functions of the organism and the vegetative regulating centers.

Through cerebral-spinal innervation, action takes place from the skin to all parts of the metamere (through transversal organization of the nervous system) and on the superior nerve centers (by the longitudinal organization of the nervous system).

Reflex massage acts on:

The brainstem: where the vasomotor center is found along with the organ-regulating centers and the respiratory centers;

The diencephalon: where the blood volume, albumins, sugar, fats, metabolism of water, sleep and allergies are regulated;

The cortex and the tuber cinereum: where the hypophysis, the neurovegetative system and the endocrine system are found.

1.4 EMOTIONAL REBALANCING

1.4.1. ERICKSONIAN THERAPEUTIC HYPNOSIS

Milton Erickson, an American psychiatrist, suffered serious health problems. He had attacks of poliomyelitis and learned techniques of self-hypnosis on his own.

He later dedicated a large portion of his life to experimenting with different hypnotic induction techniques with therapeutic purposes on his patients and on himself. He used hypnosis to allow his patients to come into contact with the resources that each one of us posses. After his death in 1980, he left humanity with a wonderful tool for change…

Hypnosis is a modified natural state of consciousness, an intermediate state between awake and sleeping that we cross through daily without realizing it (for example, when we are completely absorbed by a movie to the point that we forget what is going on around us). This is the state of consciousness that the Ericksonian therapist uses, where we can see things from a different angle, tapping into subconscious resources that are inside of us.

Ericksonian hypnosis is based on the different states of relaxation (from shallow to deep) and the active participation by the patient. Through conversation or symbolic language, the therapist guides the subconscious of the patient to enable them to find solutions to their problems.

Our subconscious, according to ERICKSON, is a grand reserve of resources, a gigantic stock of knowledge that we can use to resolve/overcome our difficulties.

The integrity and free options of the patient are completely respected by this therapy.

Ericksonian hypnosis is used in medicine and psychotherapy. It seems to be effective to free patients from certain dependencies (cigarettes, alcohol, and drugs) and to treat anxiety, sexual issues, stress, etc.

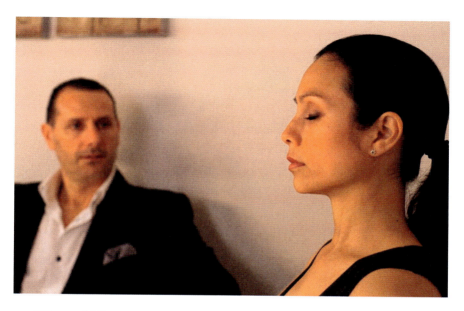

We could list many problems that can benefit from treatment with hypnosis. Generally speaking, the most frequent use is with psychologically-based problems.

"Curing with words…". Each individual is completely unique, and therefore treatment must be adapted to their uniqueness. Being a therapist means establishing a treatment that meets the needs of each patient. They must help the patient, unconsciously, to learn with "stories" (metaphors) the lessons, without having to confront realities that they are not yet ready to consciously listen to.

1.4.2 BRIEF SYSTEMIC THERAPY

Brief systemic therapy started in the 1970's in Palo Alto (California).

Brief Systemic Therapy describes "the paradoxical nature of repetitive problems".

Brief Systemic Therapy is a group of procedures and techniques that aim to help consultants (individuals, couples, families or groups) to mobilize their resources to reach their objectives in as little time as possible. It has a constructivist focus that centers on the interpersonal context of problems and their solutions, promoting active collaboration among its users.

From a historical perspective, Brief Systemic Therapy is situated between two great traditions: on one hand, the systemic tradition of analyzing phenomena in their relational context, integrating the approaches of Cybernetics, the Systems Theory or the Pragmatics of Human Communication; on the other hand, the tradition of brief therapy inspired by Milton Erickson, with his pragmatic proposal to use patient's own resources to cause change.

1.5. COMPLEMENTARY ACCOMPANYING THERAPIES.

1.5.1. PHYTOTHERAPY

The use of medicinal plants to cure is a practice that has been used since ancient times. Natural remedies, especially those that use medicinal plants, were the primary and sometimes single resource available to doctors for many years.

The applicability of phytotherapy, the use of medicinal plants, has never ceased to exist. Many of the vegetable species used for their curative virtues among ancient Egyptians, Greeks and Romans later became part of the medieval pharmacopeia that was later enriched by the contribution of knowledge from the New World.

Said medicinal plants and remedies that were used at that time are still used today.

At the beginning of the last century, the developments of chemistry and the discovery of complex processes of organic synthesis led to the new production of medicines on behalf of the pharmaceutical industry.

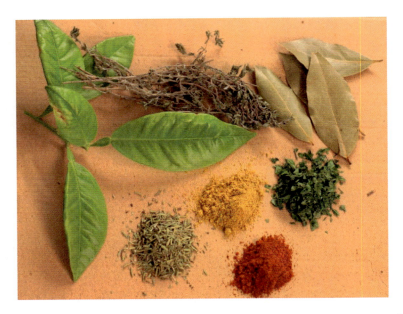

The active substances of certain medicinal plants were used to fabricate many of said medicines, with the belief that the supposed actions of said substances would increase by the possibility to carry out therapies where the amount of the active substance is greater than that possessed by the original medicinal plant in its natural state.

Nothing could be further from the trust as it has been proven that the properties of said substances were less effective and capable of causing poisoning or intolerances, which does not happen with the plant used in its natural form.

We must not forget that the plant-based remedies present an immense advantage compared to chemical treatments. In plants, active substances are biologically balanced with the complementary substances that enhance each other. This avoids their accumulation in the organism and undesirable effects are limited.

However, in spite of more research and scientific studies on medicinal plants, many of the active substances that give the plants their extraordinary qualities are yet to be understood or identified.

1.5.2. NUTRITHERAPY OR ORTHOMOLECULAR MEDICINE

Nutritherapy consists of trying to maintain or reestablish cellular equilibrium from essential elements (elements that our body cannot synthesize on its own): vitamins, trace elements, certain amino acids, polyunsaturated fatty acids.

This therapeutic approach is focused on a balanced diet. Dietary supplements are frequently added to a diet that contains one of the four varieties of the essential elements.

Nutritherapy is actually a base medicine. Nutritherapy consists of the use of the following elements:

- vitamins;
- trace elements;
- amino acids;
- polyunsaturated fatty acids.

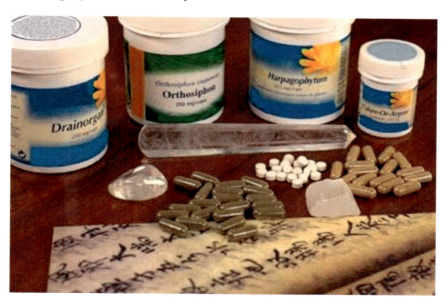

At the beginning of the century, the existence of molecules in our organism was discovered that are indispensable to life. Their deficit causes important pathological disorders, and even death if said deficit is total. What are these molecules? Basically, vitamins, trace elements, certain amino acids and polyunsaturated fatty acids. This "return to nature" has been induced by two elements:

- the development of diseases caused by medication;
- an uncontrollable fear of gigantism and eating disorders.

In chapter 1, I talked about protecting DNA and its telomeres. Here, I explain the ideal treatment for genetic repair and active maintenance of telomeres to improve health and quality of life (for 90 days):

1 gram of vitamin C per day (in the morning): repairs the plasmatic membranes and keeps cells healthy;

Vitamin E: avoids the oxidation of vitamin C and prevents its degeneration;

Omega 3: anti-inflammatory and repairs the cellular membrane;

Omega 6: controls the aging of skin;

B-group vitamins (3, 6, 9, 12): avoid the cascade of vitamins and intervenes in DNA synthesis;

Zinc: transports minerals and is involved in the metabolism of polyunsaturated fatty acids.

1.5.3. HOMEOPATHY

Homeopathy (homeos = similar; pathos = disease) is a therapeutic method that consists in giving extremely diluted doses of a substance (plant, mineral or animal) that, when administered at high doses to healthy subjects, causes similar symptoms to that of the disease.

Although this technique has been used since the time of Hippocrates, Dr. Samuel Hahnemann (1755 – 1843) was who defined the preparation and administration of these medications to activate the defenses of our organism to slowly improve or cure diseases.

Applying the laws of similarity (already established by Hippocrates), homeopathy uses the therapeutic effects of the substances, attenuating their toxicity by using very small doses that are called "infinitesimal".

The dilution process

Homeopathy defines the potency of its remedies according to the number of dilutions: more diluted substances are described as having a higher potency. The dilution process is called potentization. The potency is defined as a number where higher numbers represent greater dilution. 30X, for example, is more diluted (and therefore, according to homeopathy, more potent) than 10X.

This contrasts with conventional medicine and biochemistry where a larger quantity of an active ingredient in a medicine achieves a greater effect (positive or negative).

Some defenders of homeopathy believe that while lower dilutions have a greater physiological effect, the highest dilutions present greater effects on the mental or emotional plane.

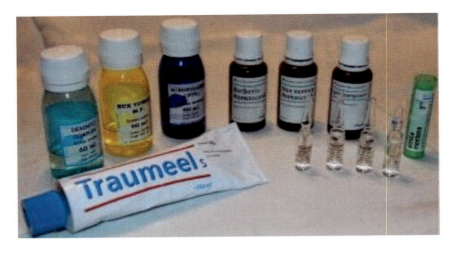

Advantages of homeopathic medicines

Homeopathy is a useful and effective therapeutic tool to treat all diseases, both acute and chronic. Sometimes it will cure while other times it will help to obtain great improvement or relief.

- Total confirmed efficacy through millions of treatments.
- Natural substances.
- Medicines with no pharmacological aggressiveness, that is, they present no side effects or contraindications.
- Apt for all types of patients: pregnant and breastfeeding women, children, elderly and diabetics.

1.5.4. HOMEOPATHIC MESOTHERAPY

Homeopathic mesotherapy is a special technique that consists of administering homeopathic medicines through the skin. Dr. Michel Pistor first described it in 1958, after randomly discovering its use when working as a rural doctor in a small French town.

The advantages of mesotherapy are summarized in an aphorism that all practitioners should keep present: "LITTLE, FEW TIMES, IN THE RIGHT PLACE".

"LITTLE" refers to the small amount of homeopathic medicine that are necessary to take advantage of their beneficial effects when administered in mesotherapy.

"FEW TIMES" refers to the low need to repeat the doses administered.

"IN THE RIGHT PLACE" expressed that homeopathic medicine that is going to be administered with the mesotherapeutic technique must be administered as close as possible to the pathology that we want to cure or improve.

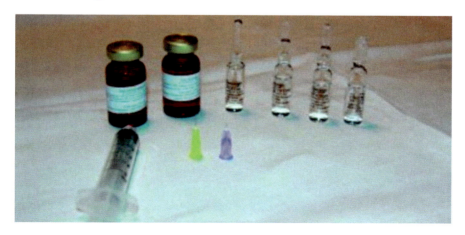

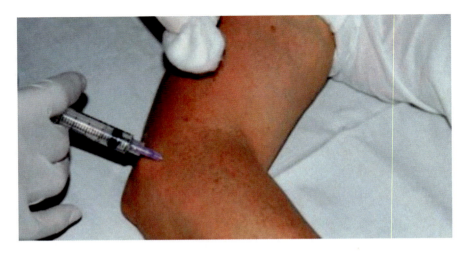

The depth to be used in mesotherapy at an intradermic level (less than 4 mm deep, as a general rule) grants mesotherapy its special characteristics and fantastic therapeutic effects.

What are the indications for mesotherapy to be used?

Mesotherapy can be indicated to treat:

- muscular and tendon pathologies;
- rheumatic, joint and bone pathologies;
- ligament pathologies;
- orthopedic pathologies and functional reeducation;
- venous disease, lymphedema;
- dermatology, acne;
- alopecia;
- hypertrophic scars and keloids.

Mesotherapy in aesthetic medicine has a very relevant role due to its contribution to the treatment of:

- wrinkles;
- lipodystrophy or cellulitis;
- skin revitalization.

1.6. ESSENTIAL OILS AND THEIR EFFECTS IN THE DAILY LIFE

D. Gary Young was one of the world's foremost authorities on essential oils. He has spent more than two decades sharing his knowledge of nature's healing powers with others, and his life's journey has helped millions transform their health and lives. For many years he directed research at the Young Life Research Clinic-Institute of Natural Medicine, validating the efficacy of essential oils and other natural healing modalities. He is the author of seven books and has co-authored four research papers published by the Journal of Essential Oil Research. He also oversees six farms on four continents, where he directs the growth, harvest, and distillation processes of the highest-quality essential oils in the world.

1.6.1. WHAT IS AN ESSENTIAL OIL?

Essential oils are subtle, volatile liquids and aromatic compounds that are distilled or pressed from plants. Essential oils are present in the oil glands, hairs, ducts, bark, stems, leaves, and flowers of many plants. They are volatile, meaning they evaporate or flash off quickly. Four types of processes are used to produce essential oils :

- Steam-distilled Oils
    - Plant material is inserted into a cooking chamber, and steam is passed through it. After the water is condensed, it is processed through a separator to collect the oil.

        - Almost all Young Living essential oils are produced through steam distillation using a proprietary low-pressure, low-temperature process.

        - Young Living's steam chambers are constructed of stainless-steel alloys to reduce the possibility of steam reacting with metal (such as aluminium or copper).

- Expressed oils

    • Are pressed from the rind of certain fruits such as tangerines, grapefruits, lemons, and oranges.

    • Rich in terpene alcohols, expressed oils are not technically essential oils, even though they are highly regarded.

    • Expressed oils should be obtained only from organically grown crops, since pesticide residues — especially highly toxic, oil-soluble, carbamate, and chloride-based petrochemicals — can concentrate in the oil.

    • Lemon (Citrus limon) is an expressed oil.

- Absolutes

    • Absolutes are essences, not essential oils.

    • They are the solid, waxy residues derived from hexane extraction of plant material, usually flower petals.

    • This method of extraction is used when the fragrance and constituents of the plant can be unlocked only using solvents.

    • Jasmine (Jasminum officinalis) and neroli (Citrus aurantium) are examples of absolutes.

- Solvent-extracted Oils

    • This extraction method uses oil-soluble solvents such as hexane, dimethylenechloride, and acetone.

- There is no guarantee that solvent residues will not remain in the finished product.

- What is a Fatty Oil?

Fatty oils are slippery oils also known as lipids. They are obtained by pressing nuts or seeds.

- They are used as carrier oils for essential oils in cooking, lotions, etc.

- They have a greasy or slippery texture.

- They are not volatile.

- Some are high in linoleic acid.

1.6.2. ESSENTIAL OILS AND FATTY OILS

A complex Chemistry…

- Essential oils contain hundreds of different chemical constituents.

- For example, lavender is composed of more than 400 different constituents, some of which are still unknown.

- Constituents often act synergistically together.

- Constituents that may be toxic in isolation are actually beneficial when accompanied by other constituents.

- The complex balance and interaction of different chemicals gives an essential oil its inherent properties. Interesting Similarity : All living things have these constituents in common:

HUMAN	PLANT
Hydrogen	Hydrogen
Oxygen	Oxygen
Carbon	Carbon
Nitrogen	Nitrogen
Sulphur	Sulphur

1.6.3. THE LIMBIC SYSTEM

How aromatic molecules influence the emotional center of the brain.

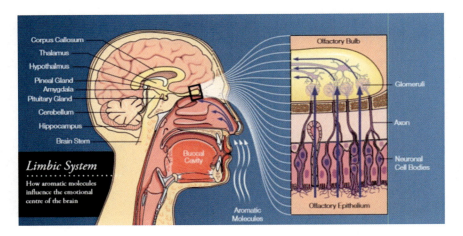

As the vapor molecules enter the nasal cavity, they are received by the receivers, something metaphorically similar to when the key is inserted into the lock. If a vapor has the correct structure (or as some say the vibration), the nerve endings receive this vapor in the form of impulse. This nervous impulse is transmitted to the limbic system.

1.6.4. HOW FRAGRANCE IS CREATED

1. Plants convert hydrogen, carbon, and oxygen into glucose.

2. Plants use minerals and nitrogen, with the help of enzymes, to convert glucose into amino acids.

3. Amino acids convert to protein.

4. Constituents with different chemical structures generate different odours.

- Mustard oil – Allyl isothiocyanate

- Garlic oil – Allyl sulfides

- Jasmine – Anthranilates

- Orange blossom – Indole

1.6.5. HOW FRAGRANCE IS REGISTERED BY THE BRAIN

1. There are two theories about scent: "lock and key" and "vibrational".

2. Lock and key suggests that as molecules within a fragrance flash into the air, they stimulate the door receptors of the olfactory system.

3. These receptors are similar to hair-like extensions of the nerve fibres that lie submerged in a thin layer of mucous.

1.6.6. ACTIONS OF ESSENTIAL OILS

- Main constituent groups :

. Phenylpropanoids:

PURIFY cellular receptors by attacking invading microbes and parasites. They purify the cell and the blood. They are able to eliminate floating free radicals from the cell and blood

There are more than 100 varieties (Eugenol / clove, mint, basil and wintergreen ...)

. Monoterpenes:

REPAIR and restore the original memory of DNA. Restart factory configuration. Essential oils can repair damaged and broken cells.

There are more than 2000 varieties (d-limonene / orange, lemon, grapefruit, balsam fir and incense ...)

. Sesquiterpenes:

DETAIL the growth of harmful cells and erase the defective information in the cellular memory. If a cell can not be repaired, the oils can stop the degeneration of the cell and eliminate it from the body so that it does not become a floating root cell.

There are more than 10,000 varieties (bisaboleno / cedar wood, sandalwood, vetiver, patchouli and myrrh ...)

1.6.7. HOW TO USE THEM

Diffuser

Young Living diffusers works as a humidifier, atomizer, and aroma diffuser in one easy-to-use product. Its ultrasonic technology breaks down any mixture of essential oils and water into millions of micro particles, which disperse in the air, and releases the components found in Young Living essential oils. The ultrasonic frequency generates waves at 1.7 million times per second, releasing molecules of essential oils in the air to help create a relaxing, spa-like environment in your home or office. It can also be used in direct inhalation (rubbing 2 drops on the palms of your hand and inhaling 4 times deep) or subtle (with necklaces or medallions to hang around your neck)

Topical application

Many oils are safe to apply directly on the skin. When applying most of the oils in children, dilute the oils with a carrier oil (15 to 30 drops of essential oil with 30 ml of good quality vegetable oil such as V6). As a general rule, when applying oils to yourself or another person for the first time, do not apply more than 2 individual oils or mixtures at one time.

Ingestion

Certain oils can be ingested, at the same time test their reactions by diluting 1 drop of essential oil in a teaspoon of a liquid such as agave, coconut oil, olive oil or rice milk.

PRECAUTIONS

Many essential oils can be used safely directly on the skin, however it is strongly recommended to dilute them in a base oil, especially in children. They should not be given to pregnant or breastfeeding women or people who take any medication without first consulting their doctor. Avoid use on skin exposed to direct sunlight as they may cause rashes or dark pigmentation.

1.6.8. « RAINDROP TECHNIQUE », A REMARKABLE REGIMEN FOR WELL-BEING

Raindrop Technique is a unique relaxation technique, combining essential oils with massage to create a truly memorable experience whilst supporting back health. It utilises a sequence of essential oils dropped on the back. Raindrop Technique can be relaxing while also supporting immune function. D. Gary Young developed the Raindrop Technique based on his research of essential oils, his knowledge of the Vita Flex technique and its reflex points on the feet, and fascinating information on the light stroking called effleurage. Anyone who has experienced Raindrop Technique is very quick to get on the massage table again to enjoy and discover new benefits of this most remarkable application of essential oils.

History of the Raindrop Technique

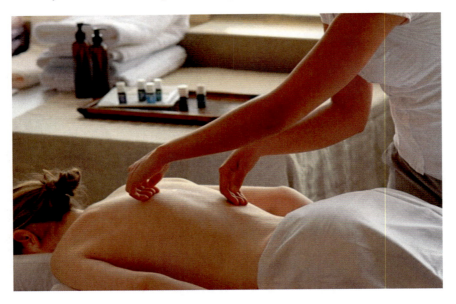

For thousands of years, medical practitioners and individuals have been using essential oils. D. Gary Young, founder and CEO of Young Living Essential Oils, has combined his vast knowledge of essential oils with the ancient energy techniques of the Lakota Indians to create the Raindrop Technique. For several generations, the Lakota Indians migrated across the Canadian border into the northern regions of Saskatchewan and Manitoba. There they often witnessed the northern lights, or aurora borealis. Those who were ill or had complicated health problems would stand facing the aurora borealis, hold their hands toward the lights, and inhale deeply. The tribal people believed that the air was charged with healing energy from the northern lights. They would mentally "inhale" this energy, allowing it to pass through neurological pathways. Many of the Lakota ancestors experienced an incredible healing effect through this process. Eventually, the Canadian borders were closed to the Lakota people, and they could no longer migrate north. Still believing in the power of the aurora borealis, they began using effleurage, or feathered finger stroking, which became associated with this healing technique. Later the Lakotas added the

practice of mentally processing energy, coupled with the light stroking, to facilitate sending this energy throughout the body. The Raindrop Technique is based on this art as developed by the Lakota Indian nation. D. Gary Young discovered that by incorporating essential oils, which are considered by Young Living to be nature's living energy, individuals could be inspired to lives of wellness, purpose, and abundance. Since its adoption in 1989, the Raindrop Technique has received an enormous amount of praise from users around the world for overall health. As a nontraditional means of addressing concerns, the Raindrop Technique has proven to be a successful alternative to more invasive remedies. Since the earliest recorded history, man has been drawn to aromatics and fragrant resins. In fact, aromatics reigned over the ancient world.

1.6.9. SOME ESSENTIALS OILS AND THEIR PROPERTIES

-**OREGANO** (Origanum Compactum):

reacting in a more aggressive manner than thyme, performs in much the same way in that it helps to stimulate the body's immune system and balance the metabolism of the body. Moreover, its use should strengthen the vitality of the body.

-**THYME** (Thymus Vulgaris):

is mainly used for its antiseptic properties. It is considered beneficial in reducing and eliminating bacteria that is present in the body. Thyme is also thought to be helpful in reducing the effects of fatigue and stress by supplying energy to the body.

-**BASIL** (Ocimum Bacilicum):

is used to relax the muscles, including those of the digestive system and heart. Plus, its use is thought to stimulate the sense of smell and reduce mental fatigue. Applied topically, basil can be used to sooth insect bites.

-**CYPRESS** (Cupressus Sempervirens):

is used to benefit the circulatory system.

Appease overflowing emotions such as sadness, impatience or irritability.

Good friend of children, calm and gives them serenity

-**WINTERGREEN** (Gaultheria Procumbens):

is used to elevate the awareness of the body's sensory system. Additionally, its use is said to relieve joint discomfort, muscle ache, and bone stress.

-**MARJORAM** (Origanum Majorana):

is utilized to calm the body's respiratory system. Its use is intended to relax the muscles and to reduce and relieve muscle spasms. Additionally, the use of marjoram is thought to calm the nerves. In short, the healing properties associated with marjoram are thought to support the proper functioning of the body's respiratory system.

-**PEPPERMINT** (Menta Piperita):

long revered for its healing properties, is used in raindrop therapy for a number of purposes. Included in these are its ability to benefit the respiratory system, sooth digestive problems, improve mental acuity, and to improve the senses of taste and smell.

CHAPTER IV

CONCLUSIONS

Ever since this protocol was launched six years ago, more than 4000 patients from all over the world have been following my method with great results for a variety of pathologies and conditions.

All of the information in this book is confirmed through daily practice.

To summarize:

- have the food intolerance test done;
- eliminate the causes and go through detoxification;
- repopulate flora and protect intestinal membrane;
- start correctly associating foods according to my philosophy;
- exercise and drink daily NINGXIA RED by Young Living.

On May 24, 2019, the Manniello Method was recognized and endorsed by UNESCO CENTER FOR TRAINING IN HUMAN RIGHTS WORLD CITIZENSHIP AND CULTURE OF PEACE

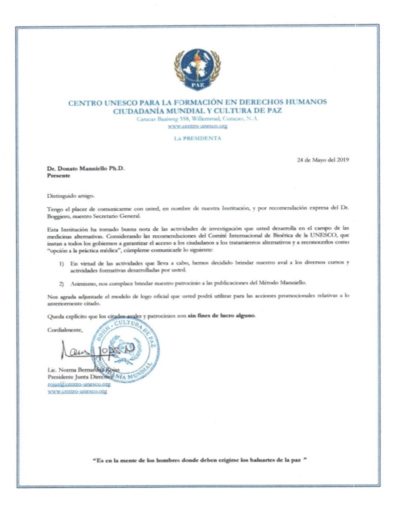

I have reached the conclusion that this is a simple and effective method. The results are quickly visible. The organism's functions are quickly recovered leading to improved well-being and tranquility, in body and mind. Energy and vitally are regained and the person that follows my method feels younger and more dynamic.

This work does not end here, but it is one step towards the never-ending search for longevity with a good quality of life.

You can imagine what will be given in the future, added to what has already been given. And all that can be created from the right to use all of one's capacities, resources, known and unknown, that are being prepared to be in your lives, your potential that will be given liberty to exist.

When one is fair to oneself, he or she discovers that they have permission to be authentic, good, and more than good…better! The happiness that we feel when we discover that each one of us has the right to be ourselves with all of our individual qualities, and that we are unique and magnificent.

There is a place in the universe that belongs to us, and we have the right to say: I am important and I have something to give to the world and receive from it. Knowing that we can open our hands not only to receive but also to give.

I hope that you hold onto this notion of discovery now and in the future. It is obviously not an obligation, but the joy to learn, the ease of learning, the pleasure of discovering that we are made to learn and that future learning can be done through pleasure. And now you can begin to understand, that there are no teachers, there are no students…there are only exchanges of experiences.

Each of us can follow our experience at our own rhythm, taking all the time needed…

If you need help, please contact me.

Thank you for reading this book!

Dr. Donato Manniello, Ph.D.

BIOGRAPHY

Doctor Donato Alberto Manniello has a degree in Osteopathy from the LUDES University in Lugano, Switzerland. His philosophy to treat patients holistically leads to a strong interest of different Alternative Medicines and he has decided to practice them exhaustively.

Dr. Manniello has been researching diet and nutrition for the last 25 years, experimenting and analyzing different nutrition methods.

With a degree in Physical Therapy (Belgium), Dr. Manniello specialized in Traditional Chinese Medicine in Paris. He has a Master's Degree in Ayurvedic Medicine, is an Expert in Health Habits (as a Health Coach), from the Official Professional Medical Association of the province of Malaga, and has an expert level diploma in Homeopathy from the Miguel de Cervantes University in Valladolid (Spain). He also specializes in food intolerances and intestinal hygiene and is a member of Slow Food International. University researcher, five years ago he creates his own method and decides to disclose it in his book "Take me with you and I will change your life". Recently, he has developed a mobile application "Manniello Method" available in 6 languages to make the knowledge of his method accessible. Trained in Young Living's "Raindrop" Therapy, directed by Tamara Packer, Dr. Donato Manniello began teaching in London and opened a series of trainings on this technique and his method across Europe. He speaks seven languages and teaches and lectures in many parts of the world, passing on his knowledge with great passion.

For more information, visit ww.manniellomethod.com

BIBLIOGRAPHY

A. Hendrickx, Les massages réflexes, Masson.

Académie de Méd. Traditionnelle Chinoise de Pékin, Précis d'acuponcture chinoise, Dangles.

ACEITES ESENCIALES, guía de referencia, sexta edición, LIFE SCIENCE PUBLISHING 2014

Albert Mosseri, La antimedicina, Mandala.

Albert Mosseri, La salud mediante la alimentación, Mandala.

André Torcque, La no medicina, el único camino hacia la salud, Mandala.

Brian Weis, Los mensajes de los sabios, Zeta.

Cáncer et alimentation, Ki.

Cic Barcelona, Curso sobre intolerancias alimentarias y salud intestinal.

Claude Haumont, Tout savoir sur l'eau, Favre.

Congelados y conservas, Ocu ediciones.

D. Merien, Ayuno y salud, Lorient.

D. Merien, Los fundamentos de la higiene vital, Puertas abiertas a la nueva era.

Danièle Starenskyj, Le mal du sucre, Orion.

David Niven, Los 100 secretos de la gente feliz, Rayo.

Deepak Chopra, Le livre des coïncidences, J'ai lu.

Diane Stein, Reiki essentiel, Guy Tredaniel.

DOSSIER SCIENTIFIQUE DE L'IFN "LES GLUCIDES" Sous la coordination de: Pr. Bernard MESSING Hôpital Lariboisière Service d'Hépato-gastroentérologie et Assistance nutritive PARIS CEDEX 10

Dr. Philippe-Gaston Besson, Acide-base: une dynamique vitale, Trois fontaines.

Dr. Alain Horvilleur, Matière médicale homéopathique, Camugli.

Dr. Claude Binet, L'homéopathie pratique, Dangles.

Dr. Frank Mirce, Oligoéléments et sante de l'homme, Andrillon.

Dr. Gabriel Contreras Alemán, Medicina naturista, Siglo XXI.

Dr. Gaspar García, Mi agenda saludable, Amat editorial.

Dr. Hay, Health Research books.

Dr. Janine Fontaine, La médecine du corps énergétique, Robert Laffont.

Dr. John Mc Dougall, Estudio sobre la mujer bantú, médico nutricionista del hospital napa de Santa Elena, California.

Dr. Kathy Bonan, Dr. Yves Cohen, Medecine orthomoleculaire, Retz.

Dr. Kousmine, Sauvez votre corps, Robert laffont.

Dr. Kousmine, Votre alimentation selon l'enseignement du Dr. Kousmine, Robert laffont.

Dr. Miguel Ruiz, La maestria del amor, Urano.

Dr. Peter Aelbrecht, Homo energeticus, Homo energeticus.

Dr. Pierre Bressy, La pratique du végétarisme, Le courrier du livre.

Dr. Robert g. Jackson, Ne plus jamais être malade, Albert Müller.

Dr. T. Colin Campbell, The China Study.

Dr. Yves Doutrelugne-Olivier Cottencin, Thérapies breves: principes et outils pratiques, Masson.

Dra. Mª Dolores de la Puerta, Protocolo Tria, Cic Barcelona.

Dra. Nieves Palacios, Dr. Luis Serratosa, Beneficios de la actividad física sobre la salud, servicio de endocrinología y nutrición del centro de medicina del deporte. Madrid.

E.Dicke-H.Schliack-A.Wolff, Thérapie manuelle des zones réflexes du tissu conjonctif, Maloine.

Eduardo Punset, Viaje a las emociones, Destino.

Étapes clé du devenir des aliments dans le tube digestif Fioramonti J. Innovations Agronomiques 36 (2014), 1-13. Département Alimentation Humaine, INRA, 180 chemin de Tournefeuille, BP 93173, 31027 F-Toulouse cedex 3

François Lelord, Le voyage d'hector, Odile Jacob.

François Roustang, Il suffit d'un geste, Odile Jacob.

Françoise Wilhelmi, El ayuno terapéutico buchinger, Herder.

Frank A. Oski, Don't drink your milk, Teach Services.

Guy-Claude Burger, La guerre du cru, Roger Faloci.

H. H. Fryette, Bases physiologiques de l'ostéopathie, Maloine.

H. H. Fryette, Principes des techniques ostéopathiques, Maloine.

Henri Laborit, Biologie et structure, Idées.

Henri Laborit, L'inhibition de l'action, Masson.

Henri Laborit, Les comportements, Masson.

Henri Laborit, Physiologie humaine, Masson.

Herbert M. Shelton, La combinación de los alimentos, Obelisco.

Hiromi Shinya, La enzima prodigiosa, Ediciones Aguilar.

Howell, Textbook of physiology.

J. Le Coz, Mesoterapia en medicina general, Masson.

Jane E. Kerstetter-Lindays H. Allen, Dietary protein increases urinary calcium, department of nutritional sciences, University of Conneticut.

Jay Haley, Stratégies de la psychothérapie, Eres.

Jean Louis Tensorer, La phytotherapie simplement, Sauramps.

Jean Seignalet, L'alimentation ou la troisième médecine, F.-X. de Guibert.

Jennifer A. Ericsson, No milk!, Harpercollins childrens books.

Jorge Bucay, Déjame que te cuente, Integral.

José Luis Parise, Casualizar, De los cuatro vientos.

Julius Mwabuki, El poder del camino al autoconocimiento, Hades.

Lynne Mc Taggart, El experimento de la intención, Sirio.

Margaret Kreig, La médecine verte, Plon.

Mark Lovendale, Quality Longevity, Pcc.

Mc Leod's, Physiology in modern medicine, Mosby Company.

Método Amaranta

Michio Kushi, Le livre de la macrobiotique, Guy Tredaniel.

Milton H. Erickson, Ma voix t'accompagnera, Homme et groupes.

Nardone et Watzlwick, L'art du changement, L'esprit du temps.

Pavlov, Progreso.

Richard Wilhelm, I Ching, Edhasa.

Robert Cohen, "Milk" the deadly poison, Argus.

Wayne W. Dyer, Accomplissez votre destinée, Carte blanche.

Wayne W. Dyer, Piensa diferente, vive diferente, De bolsillo.

William Henry Porter, Eating to live long, Bibliobazaar.

WEBS:

www.metodomanniello.com

www.youngliving.com

www.oecd.org/health/obesity-update.htm

www.who.int/features/factfiles/obesity/es/2017

www.elindependiente.com/vida-sana/2017/10/11/numero-ninos-adolescentes-obesos-se-ha-multiplicado-10-40-anos/

www.thelancet.com/journals/lancet/article/PIIS0140-6736(19)30041-8/fulltext

www.elespanol.com/ciencia/nutricion/20190404/comer-mata-personas-mundo-letal-mala-alimentacion/388211962_0.html

www.dsalud.com

www.elmundo.com

www.saludalia.com

www.fao.org

www.medynet.com

www.salusline.com

www.misfrasescelebres.com

www.ocu.org

www.who.int/topics/obesity/es/

www.cruzroja.cl

www.fongdcam.org

www.nature.com

www.unav.es

www.drcormillot.com

wikipedia.org

foro.univision.com

www.alimentacion-sana.org

Dr. Donato Manniello Ph.D.
info@metodomanniello.com
www.metodomanniello.com

Made in the USA
Lexington, KY
22 July 2019